So, That

Happened

A Memoir

CC Webster

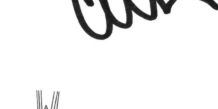

WEBSTER WORKS

New York, NY

Webster Works
www.websterworks.com
ccwebster@websterworks.com

Interior book design copyright © 2017 by Book Design Templates.
Cover design by Gus Yoo
Author photo by Carolyn Webster
Front cover image © by Africa Studio/Shutterstock
Copy editing by Stephanie Gunning

ISBN 978-0-9995413-0-2
Library of Congress Control Number 2017916305

Contents

For Matt

"Oh! I have slipped the surly bonds of Earth
And danced the skies on laughter-silvered wings."

—John Gillespie Magee, Jr.

1 THE PLAN

I was five when I decided who I wanted to be. Skipping down Park Avenue, with each jump over the seams in the sidewalk, my life in New York City revealed itself to me. On a bright winter afternoon, my family walked several yards behind me, my seven-year-old sister holding our grandmother's gloved hand and my mother's bear-like fur coat glistening in the winter air. I could hear the buckles of my father's loafers clinking with each stride as he tried to call me back from the street corner. But I wasn't paying attention to him.

To me, the city was magic come to life. My parents kept an apartment there that the family used only a few times a year, which was never enough for me. The gilded revolving front door of our apartment building spun us right out onto Park Avenue, and each time I swirled out to the sidewalk, I lit up like the city lights. Like Eloise at the Plaza, I rode up and down the elevators, greeted the doormen by name, and chatted with the little old ladies who lived in the neighboring apartments. At ninety-six, Mrs. Lowenstein in 709 had taken up Spanish lessons! Marie the maid lived in a faraway land called Queens, and Peter at the front desk wore a doorman's hat and would have his own private tea party with his flask every Friday afternoon!

I saw magic everywhere. It was in the towering buildings stretching up to the sky—I could imagine Rapunzel's hair tumbling down from the highest window of the Met Building and Prince Charming scaling hundreds of floors up from the sidewalk to rescue her. It was in the brilliantly feathered horses prancing and pulling white carriages, and the drivers tipping their top hats as they *clipped* and *clopped* past me. It was in the penguins in the Central Park Zoo that seemed to be waiting in their black-tie costumes for Mary Poppins and Bert before they exploded into a tap dance. It was in the scarlet carpet that rolled out onto the street at the Plaza Hotel, and how the jewels glittered as the ladies walked up those front stairs with their gowns trailing behind them. It was in the homeless "lost boys" sitting on the street corners; the tinkling of their coins called out for Tinkerbell and Peter Pan. I knew they were waiting for Peter because I would see him flying around town on the side of a bus. Sometimes, even Jiminy Cricket would dart across the sidewalk in front of me. It was in how the sidewalk would glitter like fairy dust under my shiny red shoes. And I would wonder how many *clicks* I had managed to get here. Like Dorothy in *Wizard of Oz*, I knew there was no place like *this*. Even when I was too small to see over the mahogany front desk in the apartment building's main lobby, I could feel the vibrating, magnetic energy of the city. Like a spell, it had me completely and irreversibly entranced.

While my family and I glided down the street on our way to a French restaurant for an early dinner, I admired the tailored sophistication of all the beautiful young women I saw stepping out of the office buildings we passed. To me, it was like watching fairytale princesses come to life in front of my very eyes. As we waited at a crosswalk, I was overcome with awe because Cinderella incarnate stood right in front of me. I knew it was she when the corners of her undone coat blew back just enough for me to catch a glimpse of her blue dress.

When Cinderella looked down and saw me staring, she smiled at me and gave me a wink with one of her perfectly shaped eyes. I couldn't even breathe, much less blink, I was so excited. My moments later, as I watched her cross the street, I took note not just of her hair, clothes, and shoes, but of how she stood tall with her shoulders squared back. She had purpose in her walk, like she was going somewhere important. I observed how one of her gloved hands gripped the handle of a briefcase as she raised the other gracefully to hail a cab. Like a dancer stepping onto a stage, she looked like she knew what she was doing and where she was going. She looked like she belonged exactly where she was and had the choreography memorized. Powerful and poised, I believed she had the world at her feet. Whereas I was just an onlooker, she looked at ease amid the bustle, like she belonged in the magic.

I was so entranced to see how, with a flick of her wrist and a tuck of her bouncy blond waves, she slid into her taxi and disappeared into the sea of lights that I decided on the spot This is who I wanted to be. This was the beginning of the plan.

Holding my father's hand as we turned the corner to the restaurant, I wondered what *my* life would be like when I was all grown up. I started imagining who I would be, where I would belong, and whether I had a say in all of it. Because if I did get to choose, I wanted to be just like that Cinderella I had seen crossing the street. I wanted to be perfect. Proud. Graceful. I wanted to walk with a purpose, like she did. I wanted to have a place in the magic. I wanted to belong in something important.

There is a moment when every child takes control of her life. It's the first time she asserts herself with the word *no,* or starts to challenge everything her parents do and say. It is a child's way of communicating individuality, of testing whether she can separate from the identity of her family. The child is looking to establish her own way of being in the world. At five years old, I was doing just that. I came to the realization that I got to choose who I would be. That I would get to design the person that I would become, and I could be anything I wanted to be. With each step over a seam in the sidewalk during that walk, I imagined my life way out ahead of me.

I loved the new life I imagined for myself. It was like I suddenly took hold of the reins instead of my father's hand. I actively imagined everything about the woman I would be and began to live into that future. My game of make-believe was invigorated by the possible reality of all that I was dreaming up. At six, I mimicked the stilettoed princess on Park Avenue by putting on my best outfit, which happened to be my sister's pink sailor suit that was delicately "borrowed" from her room.

Due to my lack of spelling capability, I scribbled the alphabet on the "desk" that was my bedspread. In focused anticipation of a business career, I played Office much more often than House or My mommy and Baby Carriage. *Just like her*, I would think to myself.

Fast forward seventeen years. I had just landed a job at one of the industry's most recognized and awarded healthcare advertising agencies and my plan was perfectly underway. At twenty-two, I marched my graduate degree straight into New York City and traded in the pink sailor suit for clothing from Barney's and Bergdorf's.

Hired right before the holidays, I couldn't wait for the manila folders, impressive lobby, and the prestige to begin. On my very first day, my high heels clicked and clacked on the marble floor as I crossed the ground floor lobby. Although it was January, my cheeks were flushed—with excitement rather than from the cold. Looking up at the high-vaulted ceiling, my nerves made me feel like I had just eaten the shrinking potion in *Alice in Wonderland.* Surely, I didn't belong with the crowd of seasoned officegoers. Would I get smaller and smaller, until my clothes were dragging behind me like a child playing dress up?

Shrinking potion or not, I gripped the handles of the structured leather bag on my shoulder and did my best to walk across the lobby with my head held high and my shoulders back, airing confidence that I really didn't have. Doing my best impersonation of someone who had held a job before, I struggled to find my place in the flow of foot traffic passing the security gates. The stream of head-phoned suits marched silently onward, like a diligent army. "Oops, so sorry," I said, as I shuffled into the procession, bumping the person in front of me.

After the checkpoint, the stream of coats divided and flowed into the double-door elevators on either side of the hall. I didn't have enough time to orient myself to the designated elevator banks for each set of floors. Caught in the stream of traffic like driftwood flowing down a rapid, I was carried to the elevator for the twenty-first through thirty-fifth floors, stopping one by one at each floor, before making it back down to the lobby where I could correct my course. I needed the eighth floor and now I was nine minutes late for orientation.

Late for my first day. A nightmare!

Once I stuffed myself into the correct elevator, I tried to appear calm though I was freaking out. *Oh my God, it's five minutes past nine and I'm late. I'm so late. I'm going get fired. Fired before I even start. And then no one will ever hire me, and I'll never get a job again. And then, I'm a failure who has to move back out of the city to live with my parents, and I'll have no friends, and no life, and no high-rise apartment with floor-to-ceiling windows, and I will die single with a bunch of cats and too many potted plants.* My anxiety level rose with the elevator and my heart pounded in my ears, matching the beat leaking out of the headphones of the guy next to me.

Ding went the elevator when it reached the eighth floor. I gripped my bag tighter, took a deep breath, and stepped out. I smoothed the front of my coat with its buttons gleaming like armor. *Be brave. Shoulders back, head up, smile. Confidence. Control. I can do this. Because this is where my life starts.*

"Good morning!" greeted a cheery receptionist without looking up. She was young enough to be right out of school, like me. I introduced myself, with a small sense of relief in feeling I could relate to this other young person in this big, marble corporate setting. But right before I let down my guard, she mechanically said, "Welcome to the agency. Orientation is waiting for you on the ninth floor."

Orientation is waiting for me. What a terrifying thought. I imagined a room full of eyes turning on me as I slowly open the door to the conference room. The speaker falls silent until I find and take my seat among the quiet, watching, waiting crowd. Then, the speaker asks me to stand and introduce myself and then tell the room "a fun fact about me." Horror. Simply horror.

I opened the door to the orientation room to find a room full of just-graduated twenty-somethings seated behind desks and listening to the human resources director teach them about timesheets. I get a quick nod and "a come on in" from the director and took my seat. No turning eyes, no silence. No fun facts. *Okay, not so bad.*

As the director moved on to the explanation of payroll, I looked to my right and saw a painted mural of a tree on the wall, stretching from floor to ceiling, like the one we had in kindergarten. Each of the tree's branches was designated to a different department of the agency, and the branches' leaves were filled with headshots of the heads of those departments. My inner five-year-old was thrilled to be coddled and she began excitedly mapping out her journey to the top of the tree, swinging like a monkey from branch to branch.

In my first few weeks at the agency, I arose with excitement every morning. I couldn't wait to get to the office. My plan was in full swing, and I was determined to build a place and a purpose for myself. I was determined to belong in something important. I laid out my clothes every night with great care. I would eagerly wait by the office delivery door at 4 AM to pick up the breakfast catering for the 9 AM morning meeting, ensuring the food was meticulously set up and ready on time for the meetings that I stood outside the doors of. As I shifted my weight from one heeled foot to the other, I would wait hours for the printer to cough up hundreds upon hundreds of pages of *reference packs,* a term that was a mystery to me at the time but kept me printing and filing late into the night. I made sure the Diet Coke labels were all turned to the outside when I stacked them in sets of six in the boardrooms, and I would have the black pens and crisp paper pads precisely positioned at each place setting on those long mahogany tables. I was driven to be perfect, and do everything *perfectly.* I only sometimes would question my college degree when working around the clock booking travel, waiting on hold for hours on end to confirm an aisle seat, and then finding a twenty-four-hour FedEx office from which to ship printed copies of the travel itinerary.

My intense drive to belong in my new corporate world did get me attention at the agency in those early days. My boss at the time loved to page me on the booming office intercom, just to watch me come hurtling around the corner with a pile of folders flapping in my arms as I sprinted to his office in my dress and heels. I started early, and I stayed late, hell bent on proving myself. I was desperate to be in control of where I would go and who I would become.

Everything had to be perfect, because I had it all planned out.

After eight years with the agency, I had gone from New York to London and back, working my way across the different departments of the agency's network. During my year in London, I launched global ad campaigns for the agency's top-tier pharmaceutical company clients, all while immersing myself in British culture. This took a million pints of lukewarm beer, and countless nights of singing karaoke across the city with my office mates. In London, I drank copious amounts of tea, wrote flowery and extremely polite emails, and apologized well beyond proportion. My ambitious New York work ethic was a contrast to the local ethos. When I stayed late working on a presentation the night before a big new business pitch to a company in Paris, my team thought I had simply lost my mind as they all trotted to the pub at five o'clock. *Who else was going to do it? Our slides had to be PERFECT!* "Don't worry guys, I've got it," I told them.

Back in New York, I continued to rise through positions and promotions. The higher I rose, the more I felt that I was in the right place doing the right thing. The more I felt like I had a purpose. In addition to the growing list of accolades from senior management, I was proud of what I was doing during the day. To me, I was bringing groundbreaking medicine to those that needed it. The pharmaceutical giants were working to save lives, and I was a part of that mission. A true believer, I watched the advancements of science and research come out of these companies and knew I had helped shape the ways it touched the world. I lived surrounded by medicine, technological advances, and breakthrough therapies. I saw how many problems we could solve and how many lives we could change, all with once-a-day pills. Gathering in those boardrooms with my colleagues, I felt more and more like I belonged in the swirling magic of it all. The ad campaigns, the media plans, TV spots, all of it. The life I had planned since childhood was well underway, and the person I wanted to be was coming to life.

Now, at twenty-nine, I had been selected to join an elite team in the agency. My meetings were filled with CEOs, presidents, and managing partners. I worked long days in high-stress situations with people with enormous egos (mine included). Every day I was putting everything I could into not just keeping my career on track, but accelerating it forward.

After one exceptionally long day spent in the agency's war room, which is a large boardroom that serves as a sort of club house for the executives, I was packing up my laptop to head home. After sixteen straight hours in the room that is reserved for the "When Shit Gets Serious" my moments, the chairs were finally empty, and I could breathe. It was

February. Looking out the windows that overlooked Forty-Second Street, I could see snow falling through the city lights. I could see my reflection in the dark glass. My long blond hair fell loosely around my shoulders, and as I put on my coat to adjust it the woolen collar grazed my neck. I realized that I had been scratching my neck and chest throughout the day. *Ugh. Not again. It's irritated with that same rash. I'll just take an antihistamine when I get home. And maybe put on that steroid cream the dermatologist gave me. That seemed to work last time.*

Once I packed up, I walked through the marble lobby and out onto the street to hail a cab. I piled myself into the cab that pulled up to the curb, taking notice of my achy muscles as I slid into the back seat. *Didn't realize standing all day was a total body workout. Great, no gym tonight. Two Advil should fix it.*

During the ride downtown, I checked my calendar for tomorrow's schedule and starting planning for the next day's meetings as Park Avenue whizzed by. The snow had already covered the ground by the time I got out of the taxi and went into my building ten minutes later. I shivered as I crossed out of the cold. *Should have worn more layers,* I mused.

I opened the door to my apartment and was greeted by another view of the sparkling city skyline through the windows. After basically running a daycare center for the managing partners and president of the agency, I was too tired to make dinner and ordered sushi instead. My usual order arrived a short twenty minutes later, which always makes me feel uneasy, like the California and spicy tuna rolls might have been premade hours before. Despite my speculation, I scarfed down a few bites with half a bottle of red wine and watched mind-numbing reality TV. I looked at the remaining nine pieces of sushi left on the plate before I threw it in the garbage. *Why am I not hungrier? I usually eat two full rolls. Well, I guess I did have a full sandwich today in the boardroom. I'm probably still full.* The rolls hit the bottom of the garbage bin with a thud.

When I could barely keep my eyes open any longer, I brushed my teeth, took the Advil, the antihistamine, smothered my itchy neck in white, sticky steroid cream, checked my email one last time, and headed to bed. Even though I was exhausted from the day, I found myself lying awake in the dark to plan my upcoming meeting with the managing partners of my agency.

As with every meeting that I led, I saw this meeting as a chance to prove myself, earn my seat at the mahogany table of the agency, and keep my career moving full speed ahead according to my plan. With each promotion, the stakes had gotten higher and there was even less room for *failure,* a word that made me feel nauseas. Laying in my bed, tired muscles aching, I tossed and turned as I planned the meeting. As my imagination ping-ponged me back and forth from shattering failure to shimmering success, I fell into a restless sleep only to be awoken a few hours later at 3 AM covered in sweat. *Premade sushi. I knew it. Those overpriced pirates. Never ordering from them again. I'll write a scathing Yelp review in the morning.*

I kept sweating throughout the early hours of the morning. Perspiration dripped down my chest and back, drenching my old, torn tee shirt. *Aside from the sushi, I'm probably stressed out. Nothing a Xanax can't solve.* And off to sleep again as the little white tablet slid down my throat.

That night I dreamed of myself as a little girl skipping in her red shiny shoes down Park Avenue.

2 A Wingnut, a Rhino, and a Surgeon Walk into a Bar

In the next few weeks, the rash, the fatigue, the aches, the chills, and the night sweats continued to get worse. As they did, I became more and more dedicated to inventing and assigning reasons for each symptom to exist, including every possible cause from stress and exhaustion to the wrong detergent. Since I was running out of fresh turtlenecks that would hide the rash on my neck from my colleagues, that was the symptom I Googled first.

Based off the countless images online showing severely pocked necks, throats, and collarbones, I decided that I could have one the following diseases: poikiloderma of civatte (a pus-filled bubble), *Tinea versicolor* (a pernicious yeast), *Lichen simplex chronicus* (rough skin caused by repeated rubbing), *Pityriasis rosea* (a disgusting red patch with a raised border), or just run-of-the-mill atopic dermatitis. I latched on to the last one because it didn't sound like a spell out of Hogwarts, and my well-trained imagination quickly served up an explanation to support. *Ah ha! That's it! Nailed it. I switched my laundry and dry-cleaning place a few weeks ago, so obviously the harsh chemicals in the electric blue gooey detergent is "atopically" irritating my "dermis."*

While in the office, I silently fought through the fatigue and the aches and continued to run meetings at full pace with every ounce of energy I had. As I dragged my fatigued self through my long, busy days, I knew that I couldn't falter in those boardrooms. I had worked too hard to get there. There was too much to lose. There was my reputation, my position, and my status to uphold, and once the partners smelled fear, I was terrified that their trust in me would be forever broken.

This chainmail of confidence that I had built link by link was getting heavier and harder to hold up, but overall, I considered my gallant efforts to keep going despite how shitty I felt successful until one of the senior vice presidents pulled me aside to ask if I was okay. She said I looked very, very pale.

"What? Noooo, I'm just from the North," I said with a laugh. Humor, self-deprecation, and sarcasm always being my go-to moves when things got awkward. "This is my natural shade of paste. It's a winter white. I'm fine!" *Liar, liar pants on fire.*

Turtlenecks, mock necks, and silk scarves all covered the evidence of the rash. You see, a blotchy neck might be mistaken for nerves, which I was sure would ruin everything I had worked for in one, red swipe. Like sharks smell blood or wolves sense fear, the executives seemed as if they could sense the weak. I was afraid that once I showed one flaw, any flaw, the illusion of my competence was over. Coded as "not the right fit," me and my work would be passed on to the next team of executives, without hesitation.

You see, I understood and respected the process of moving personnel around, fully and completely. It was this very corporate culture that I had learned to so swiftly navigate. I understood. The stakes were always high, the timing always tight, and the executives needed the best. The best person for the job was confident. The best could solve anything. And the best never faltered.

I was scared to show my nerves to a room full of CEOs, managing partners, and senior VPs would mean that they saw me as unprepared or incapable. From this perception of weakness, one could never recover. The tarnish could not be wiped clean. I had worked so hard to fit in, to earn my seat at the table, to be heard, and to be valued. So, if it took a turtleneck to shield myself in the war room, I was happy to trot over to the GAP to clean out their inventory.

Well, the turtlenecks, Advil, and coffee began to fail me. My symptoms were intensifying. By midafternoon, the aches would fully take over. On night's when there was deadline, we'd be working work late. My eyes would glaze over at midnight while staring at the graphic designer's screen as we made last-minute changes to the presentation slides for the next day. I looked pale and shaky, and had lost a lot of weight. One day, I had to use a binder clip to hold my pants up, and as I reached to the top of the presentation screen I noticed that one of the graphic designers had caught a glimpse of the shiny clip. And so, to the doctor I went.

This general practitioner of mine was a total wingnut. I had picked her out of the hat that was my insurance-approved list of providers. Her office was two blocks from mine, and the staff always seemed to be able to find me last-minute appointments, should I have a stye, a nasal infection, or a urinary tract infection. This covered all that I really needed, especially since my annual blood work only ever came up with a slight vitamin D deficiency.

I sat in the waiting room alongside a group of workers comp seekers. These men looked like construction

I said no to both offers. Needing Botox injections would mean that I was old, which I clearly wasn't yet! And taking a mood stabilizer was just weird! I was not unstable! Was I? That wouldn't suit the life script I had written on Park Avenue. I was the perfect shiny princess hailing a taxi.

This time my pharmaceutically inclined doctor listened with dramatic sympathy to my symptoms and then drew blood. She told me she suspected the Epstein-Barr virus, aka mononucleosis, which four days later would be confirmed by the blood test she ran. "Okay, honey . . . ," she said. She always called me *honey* or *sweetheart,* like an old person. Actually, she'd had so much work done on her face that I really couldn't tell her age. The top of her face was thirty and the bottom was sixty-five, so let's average it out at forty-seven and a half. "Although to be honest, you are a little old for mono, I want you to take these." She handed me a bottle of horse pills. "If these don't work after a week, I'd like you to go see a specialist to rule out other things . . . like lymphoma."

Okay, crazy lady, I thought. Then I took the pills and ran the two blocks back to the office desperate to make my two o'clock meeting with the partners.

After a week of choking down those pills, which were the size of miniature ponies, the symptoms persisted. A specialist, the wingnut had said. *What kind of specialist? Should they be special in fatigue, aches, night sweats, or rashes? So many problems, so many options. I don't even know what I have. It would be my luck to need a very rare specialist. One that doesn't exist at all. Or perhaps they would be exceptionally rare, like a unicorn, and the only one is somewhere weird, like in Iowa. And I don't have time to go to Iowa. And I will have to suffer like this for the rest of my life.* Panic on the dancefloor.

Since I had always been healthy, I had never really felt the need to research doctors before. I just took the first one available. And if I really had a problem, my mother usually got involved and sorted it all out for me. I would end up with an appointment time and an address. "Don't forget to bring your insurance card," my mother would say, as if I was a nincompoop.

In this case, with my mother not yet involved, I called Dr. Wingnut's office and got a referral to see this "specialist." Special in what way I did not know. There were a few red flags. The doctor said it was her "friend" who "should be able to take you immediately." Wouldn't any friend of a wingnut be a wingnut? And could he be *that* good if his schedule was gaping open? *Where are all your patients?* I brushed my concern aside for the sake of time, made an appointment, trusting Dr. Wingnut's word, since I had a TON of work to do.

As promised, the mystery specialist had an opening that week and I headed right in, again, right in the middle of a crazed workday. As I arrived for my appointment, the frosted glass door of the midtown medical office read: ENT, Sinus Surgery, Rhinology. *Ah ha . . . That's interesting. Okay, maybe I have a lingering sinus infection? That's what it is. Here we go.*

Despite my intensifying symptoms, this second doctor's visit was so far from my priority list. As usual I was frantically glued to my email in this new waiting room, trying to keep a project moving along at warp speed. I was supremely annoyed that my appointment was running twenty minutes late and I couldn't wait to run back to the office like a golden retriever runs back to its owner with a stick. *Did you miss me?!*

After I sat tapping my foot, refreshing my email, and waiting in anticipation to get this over with, I was finally called in to Dr. Rhino's office. *About damn time.* His office was clean and white, with few unrecognizable instruments on the sterile counter. Those instruments were thin, long, and hooked, which made me feel uneasy. I sat in the exam chair and repeated my symptoms just as I had done with Dr. Wingnut, and he listened patiently.

As any well-prepared patient does, I rattled off possible causes and illnesses I had harvested from WebMD earlier that week, after the mono idea had been squashed. Considering the aches, fatigue, night sweats, rash, and weight loss, my self-diagnosis had chalked up my condition as a combination of simply stress, a thyroid imbalance, and hormonal fluctuations, all with a side of atopic dermatitis. Pleased with my own preparedness, I said, "So, doctor, what do we think?" as if we were in this together.

I'm always impressed with myself when I self-diagnose in the doctor's office. As I'm rattling off Latin words and showing off my deep understanding of mechanisms of action and the intricacies of the human body, I am helping the doctor do his job, and he soon sees me not as a patient, but a *partner*. I like to imagine he thinks to himself, *Now THIS is how my appointments should go. This patient gets a gold star. We can work together. She speaks my medical language—maybe she can help me solve the mystery. This will be fun!*

"Well, let's take look-see, shall we?" he answered mechanically, giving me the feeling he was waiting for me to finish and wasn't as impressed with me as I was.

Dr. Rhino stuck a so-called "tiny" camera down my nasal passage to take a little tour of my paranasal sinuses, my pharynx, my larynx, my torus tubarius, my arytenoid cartilage, and my lymphoid circus. If you're wondering how I know all these fancy words, remember I was in advertising for the pharmaceutical industry for eight years. With makes me think that I'm practically a Ph.D.

With the exception of telling me to cough, the doctor was silent as he probed around in my face and hauled the tiny camera out of my nose like a fisherman with a net full of fish. In this case, it felt like a net full of swordfish, a couple piranhas, and some spikey blowfish, but that's neither here nor there. Then he stood back against the wall, shrugged his shoulders, and shook his head. "I don't see anything out of the ordinary, other than a few swollen glands," he said. "This is normal for a little virus and should go away on its own. Overall, it looks fairly normal."

WHAT?! Normal?! No, no, no, sir. No infection? That can't be. I am so tired I could fall asleep standing. I am so achy, it's like I shattered my bones with a hammer. And I CANNOT wash my sheets one more time or I will scream. Forget the rash. The night sweats are killing me. I don't even care about the rash anymore. I'll just wear turtlenecks forever, even in the summer. Like Diane Keaton. You just have to fix me! You must know what this is! There's no "not knowing" allowed! I can't go on like this!

"But, doctor," I said, "something is definitely wrong with me." I spoke with urgency as I hushed my inner child's tantrum. "What about my thyroid? My mother had thyroid problems. Or my hormones? I read that imbalanced hormones can cause night sweats. Like in menopause! Right? Maybe I'm perimenopausal? We have to figure this out!" I wasn't leaving without a next step. I wanted an answer.

Despite my obvious desperation, Dr. Rhino told me he couldn't think of anything else to do other than recommend me to his brother, who was "an endocrine surgeon and . . ." (I heard) "ozarktripodbellsandwhistlesologist" who was "better at the thyroid and the hormone stuff.

"I am more of a nose guy," Dr. Rhino said with a note of defense.

An endocrine and a what?! "Okay, great. Let's do that," I said calmly. I tried to keep my frantic anguish concealed by looking contemplative and nodding my head, as if I concurred with the assessment and the referral.

Dr. Rhino texted his brother right then as I sat in the exam chair. He confirmed my appointment for the next week, shook my hand, said, "Good luck," and sent me on my way.

It was at this point where the frustration of not feeling well began to turn to fear of illness. *How many more doctors will I need to see before one of them can diagnose this? How mysterious is this disease, if it IS a disease? The symptoms are getting worse every day. How much worse are they going to get? How will I do my job and hold up my life when I can barely get out of bed? Something is very wrong with me. I need help.*

For this next visit, I took a whole different approach. This was getting serious. I researched the brother, Dr. Surgeon, and I found that, different from

Dr. Rhino, Dr. Surgeon specialized in specific diagnoses and surgeries. Thyroid diseases, thyroid cancers, head and neck tumors, head and neck cancers, adenoid cystic carcinoma, laryngeal cancer, mucoepidermoid carcinoma, and squamous cell cancer to be precise. They all flooded the screen of my laptop with overwhelming abundance. You would think this list would throw me into panic, making me think I had each and every one. Well, it didn't. Each time carcinoma or cancer jumped out of the list, I immediately dismissed them as I read them. *That wouldn't happen to me.*

There I was again, in another waiting room, anxiously refreshing my email, however this time, the anxiety was twofold. On one hand, I feared another failed doctor's visit, and another "everything appears fairly normal" analysis. *Where would I go next? How long can I cycle through these disappointing visits? Something is very wrong!*

On the other hand, I was sitting in a neck surgeon's waiting room. My mind started spinning. *Maybe this is serious. Maybe I will need some sort of surgery. Or maybe I have multiple sclerosis. My grandmother had that. Or it is my thyroid. Maybe I will need to get it removed. I hate surgery. Not to mention, I would have a big scar on my neck. I would need to take time off work. Oh god. My job. Shit.*

A few minutes later, propped up in Dr. Surgeon's exam chair, I recited the symptoms yet again. This time, I really leaned in to the self-diagnosed thyroid disease, offering up my mother as the blame. Dr. Surgeon listened patiently until I was finished, then he looked me straight in the eye and asked, "Can I be honest with you?"

"Yes," I said, in a squeaky voice, disarmed by his seriousness.

"I think you have Hodgkin lymphoma."

I stared at him blankly. Then, out of some cavernous ravine deep inside me, erupted tears. They burst out of me like water from a geyser. I immediately thought I was dying. And with good reason. My uncle had died of non-Hodgkin lymphoma a decade earlier, at forty-seven, alone in his sleep.

And it all played out before me. I was a child when Uncle Johnny went bald. He would tie a red bandana on his head in the winter, and when asked to play with us, he would say, "Not today, girls, Uncle John isn't feeling very well."

I was too young to understand what cancer was, but I had seen lots of bald men put sunscreen on their heads at the first tee. To me, it was no big deal. But around Uncle Johnny, and being told he was sick, I watched the adults for signs of what to say, when to laugh, and more importantly, when not to laugh. This was exceptionally difficult when he made jokes about his own bald head and his shocking resemblance to Uncle Fester from the Addams Family. He would use humor to deflect the disease, which confused me at the time.

Even through his sick years, Uncle Johnny was big and boisterous, always the life of the party. He knew how to laugh and tell a good, roaring story at the dinner table. He died ten years later eighty pounds lighter and with yellowing skin and gaunt circles under his eyes. You could hardly have recognized him.

Dr. Surgeon didn't realize he was telling me my fate was the same as Uncle John's. He was telling me that I had cancer, that I was going to wither away and suffer, and that I was going to die in ten years. Which was definitely not enough time for my life plan to unfold. In the exam chair, I cried for the children I wouldn't have, I cried for my parents who would host my funeral, and I cried for the life that I had lost.

As I tried to take control of the swells of tears, I said to Dr. Surgeon, "But we don't know that yet, right? We have to test, right?!" And I exposed my neck, prompting any sort of test, not caring if he sliced me open right then and there.

"Yes, we will test, but I am very sure." *Stop telling me that I'm going to die! At least have the death certificate come from one of these machines in here! Or a lab test! Don't we need a lab test?! Some sort of proof?! You only have a theory! You are guessing! All*

*of you doctor people have been wrong, so I want to
see hard evidence! Oh my god, I am going to die.*

And we did the liquid biopsy right there, as I sat
quietly crying in the exam chair, gripping its cold
leather arms. The needle the size of a turkey baster
went in to my neck, poked around, came out, and
went off to the lab with the afternoon mail.

As Dr. Surgeon opened the exam room door to the
waiting room, he said, "I'll call you tomorrow at two
o'clock when the results come in. Hang in there, we
will know for sure tomorrow."

I apologized for the tears as I awkwardly maneu-
vered myself off the exam chair, which reclined like a
dentist's chair I literally slid off from mid-operation
when I had my tonsils removed. Then I joked that he
would probably need a mop for the damage, and Dr.
Surgeon smiled sympathetically, recognizing my desperate attempt to lighten the situation, patted me on
the shoulder, and sent me home.

As one can imagine, the most difficult thing I had
to do after leaving Dr. Surgeon's office that night was
to switch out of the mode of "I'm going to die in a few
years" and switch into the mode of "I need to prepare
for tomorrow's meeting." Life kept rambling on and I
had to keep up.

When I told Matt and my parents about the doctor's visit that night, I was reassured that nothing was
confirmed yet, Dr. Surgeon could be wrong, what

Johnny had was different anyhow, and that either way, we are getting closer to fix whatever problem I was having. My father chalked the mandated next step up to an easily excitable and profit-driven healthcare system fear-mongering me in to doing more tests and biopsies and such. My father went on for about for thirty minutes, blowing off steam.

As ultrasounds and biopsies swirled my thoughts, I tried to focus on tomorrow's meeting schedule.

I sat at my counter at home preparing my notes for the next day's meeting. I had spent countless hours over the past four weeks preparing everything I could think of to impress the partners. I felt like had to bring new ideas to the table, and make sure I had an answer for every question. I had worked so hard to get where I was. The stakes were high, and I could not fail.

While looking over my notes one by one that night, I forced myself to ignore the alarm bells that were blaring in my head. I pushed the idea of cancer, of death, of Uncle Johnny away. Buried it deep. I didn't even Google what Dr. Surgeon had said. I justified ignoring it to myself. *That would only send me down a rabbit hole and it would freak me out. It would be like that time that I read the medical dictionary in the middle school library. Every symptom seemed easily relatable and, BAM, I had early onset Alzheimer's disease in sixth grade. I thought I had everything after reading that damn book.*

But fear kept oozing its way back in and I had to keep taking it by the hand, coax it back upstairs, and tuck it into bed like a child who can't sleep. *This is just a bad scare. Like an abnormal pap smear. All of a sudden, with one swipe of the cotton swab, you think you have cervical cancer and then oopsie daisies, you don't. Everything is fine, they say. We will see you next year, they say. It is just a bad scare. Don't worry. Dr. Surgeon will call tomorrow and we will finally know what is wrong. And it won't be cancer. And if it is . . . it won't be. Don't even think about that. But if it is . . . Night, night. Don't let the bed bugs bite.*

So, there I was the next day, Wednesday at 2:18 PM, waiting for my cancer call as I led my meeting with the managing partners in the war room. To them, this was without a doubt just another pitch and just another meeting, but to me, it was my moment. Dressed in all black, I stood at the front of the room. *Shoulders back, head up.* I took notice of how often each of them would reach for their phones. As I kept taking them through the plan of action for the pitch, I tried to pick up speed, like the timer was ticking on my audience, and soon they would burst out of their gates like horses to a field. I feared that I'd lose them to start the swirl of chaos that comes with seven different, often opposing, and frantic opinions of how it all should go. I had to keep order. I felt like I had to keep control over the room.

And right then, in the middle of my sentence, my phone rang. It buzzed and vibrated on the wooden conference room table. And I recognized the number on the screen. I had been waiting for that number, yet I considered letting the call go to voicemail so as not to interrupt that my moment, *my* moment. But the wave of anxiety that was triggered was too deep and it soon took over.

"I'm so sorry, I *have to* take this call," I said apologetically to the table of partners. "I will be right back; it will just be a second."

I had never stepped out of a meeting in my life and the walk from the front of the room to the back was long and silent, as the executives seemed to look at each other across the table. Looking back now, I'm sure they didn't mind getting a quick break to check their emails, but it killed me to walk out.

Once huddled next to the stacked chairs in the dark closet outside of the war room, I took the call.

"Your liquid biopsy test came out negative," Dr. Surgeon said to me. And just as I finished processing the word *negative,* he continued, "but I think it is a false negative. I have booked you in for a surgical biopsy tomorrow at three o'clock. I strongly recommend we do this. I still believe you have Hodgkin lymphoma. Can you make it tomorrow?"

This last remark did not sound like a question.

"Yes. Yes, three o'clock tomorrow," I said automatically, despite knowing the next day's back-to-back meeting schedule. I would just have to cancel. "This time we are going to find out what this is, right?" I asked desperately. Fear had taken me over.

Dr. Surgeon reassured me that the surgical biopsy would tell him exactly what was going on, and then we would "go from there."

To me, "going from there" meant two things. The first was planning my march to death with a cancer diagnosis, and the second was continuing to make more appointments, see more doctors, all while withering away due to my now debilitating symptoms, with no cause and no cure. Which would be worse, I couldn't tell.

I hung up the phone. The front of conference room door was smooth and white. I could feel my breath bounce off its sheen as I stood there with my hand on the cold metal push panel. As Forty-Second Street buzzed beneath me, I took a deep breath and closed my eyes. I smoothed my silk shirt. It was like I was carefully putting my armor in place, piece by silver piece.

One, two, three, push.

I walked back into the war room to resume my post like nothing had happened.

3 OOMPA-LOOMPA DOOMPETY DOO

Everything was happening so fast, it was hard to digest it all. The doctor's visits, the ultrasound, the biopsy, the surgery appointment. It felt like the tea cup ride gone wrong at a fair. I was swirling, and swirling again, while the world blurred away around me, out of control. I held on to the center bar with all my strength just trying to keep myself from flying out of my seat, out into oblivion. My entire body was braced and even though my knuckles were white and my muscles ached with exhaustion, I held on. With every ounce of my being, I held on.

When I turned up at the hospital for my surgical biopsy the next day at 2:45 PM, I was greeted by a bill with a smiling southern lady at the other end of it. "'Hi, sweetheart. Checkin' in? Great, there you are. Cash or charge?" she said with a sweet southern drawl, like I was checking into a cozy bed and breakfast. Her vocal tone easily could have made me mistake the whopping hospital bill that was placed in front of me for a plate of warm biscuits, fresh out of the oven.

Relieved that my credit card didn't combust into flames as she swiped a few thousand dollars on it, I took a seat in the waiting room. *What's money at a time like this,* I thought. Then I recognized the genius of the hospitals for leveraging that very moment when their patient throws their wallet to the wind. From a marketing perspective, it's brilliant. Get 'em while they're vulnerable.

Matt, my now-husband and then-boyfriend, had come with me that day. I held his arm as he tried to distract me with stories about myself. This typically works every time, but that day was a struggle. "Here we are again," he said with an affectionate smile as he squeezed my hand.

"It's definitely been a series of unfortunate events," I replied with a laugh. It really was the no-good, terrible, horrible, very bad *year.*

This was not the first surgery that Matt and I had experienced together. A year to the day prior, we had been skiing in Vermont. It was our last run on our last day, and I had insisted we go out of bounds to get the fresh snow. As we *swooshed* through the sludge that is what Vermont calls powder, I heard Matt yell from behind me, "MOOSE!" As an avid nature fan and large animal lover, I was only slightly concerned about the size of the antlers on this thing, and whether we had skied over its baby. So, I turned around to try and catch a glimpse of the beast while I was mid swoosh, and then *POP.* It was a deep, explosive, strangely satisfying sound, like a champagne cork as it blasts out from the bottle. I buckled immediately and planted my ass in the snow. *Uh oh.* Matt skied down to me to see what happened.

"What happened?!" I repeated back angrily, immediately blaming him for my fall. "You said you saw a moose! What moose?! I don't see a moose!" I was even more annoyed that there was no moose.

"No! I said that I had to tighten my BOOTS," he replied.

As he tried to help me up, my right leg gave way and back down I went, into the wet snow. "Ouch ouch ouch, that felt weird," I said. "It feels like my knee bones are running into each other."

"Wait a minute, did that sound come from your leg?" Matt asked with disbelief, taking a step back to analyze the situation.

"You heard that?" He was one hundred yards behind me, and was wearing a helmet, which is a testament to the loudness of the popping sound my leg made.

"Uh, yeah. . . . It wasn't your . . . Oh no! Was that your knee? Does it feel wiggly?" he asked cautiously. He had torn his ACL in high school, so immediately recognized what had happened.

Still in denial, I contradicted him. "No. It's not my ACL. No, no, no. I just pulled something. Just hyper-extended it. See look, I'm fine," I told him as I flopped my heavy boot around in the air and winced. "And my knees are always wiggly, because I'm extremely flexible. It's not my ACL," I said with a scoff, still annoyed that he had made me fall.

Other than my knee bones colliding with each other, there was only a slight ache—and it quickly subsided, which I took to mean that I was fine. How-ever, each time I tried to stand up, the whole leg gave out. I even tried a turn or two on my one good leg to see if I could get down the hill, but I kept floundering around like a baby bird out of its nest.

On my fifth failed attempt to stand, Matt was now in full survival mode, whereas I was continuing to in-sist that "I can do it." He had realized we were stranded mid-mountain and out of bounds on a closed trail, with no way to get down. The only way to go was back up the mountain, and we were hundreds of yards from the top. We couldn't even *see* the top. "That's it. I'm going to get help. I'll be back as fast as I can. Don't move," he said as he clicked out of his skis. But with his first step up the mountain, his boot sunk three feet into the snow. One step, sink. Another step, sink. It took him ten minutes to traverse ten feet.

"How's it going?" I asked guiltily as I watched him struggle those first ten feet. The mountain seemed to get bigger and steeper with each of his steps.

"Fine," he said without turning around. "Just don't move." Despite the agonizing effort of each step, Matt kept going at the lumbering speed of a tranquilized bear and eventually got smaller and smaller looking as he climbed up the mountain, until he disappeared over the ridge at the top.

While I waited for him to come back with the ski patrol, I tried to enjoy the view. I was sitting in the middle of nowhere, surrounded by snow and trees, without a soul in sight. This wasn't terrifying, it was *beautiful*, I tried to convince myself. It was one of those clear, crisp blue-sky days and I could see forever. The blue was just about to start turning to yellow and orange and I settled in to watch the light show as the day faded away behind the mountains. Every now and then, I tried to test out my knee to see if it miraculously had healed itself, but the bones would crunch together, and it gave out again and again. I came around to realize that Matt was right. I knew it was my ACL. The lower half of my leg felt detached, and

I was familiar with the injury from my sister's experience.

Shit. Well, at least my story is better than hers. I was skiing, and she was jumping over people in college. But shit. I can't believe this happened to me. I'm too flexible for this to happen. Shit. I will need to have surgery. Shit. I'm going to have to take time off work. And, I'll have to go on that machine that moves my leg. Shit. So much physical therapy.

It was in moments like these that I habitually would try to turn a situation on its head. I reluctantly tried to coach myself into the idea that shit happens that's out of my control and I just have to deal with it, which is an idea that has never come naturally to me. It is so unnatural, in fact, that I find the pessimistic side of my brain quick to argue with the optimistic side, and my brand of pessimism always wins.

As the bickering in my head was just starting and anxiety was binding my chest, I heard the growl of the ski patrol snowmobile coming towards me and breathed a sigh of relief.

While I was getting tucked in to the long, red sled at the back, Matt hovered over me, making sure I was buckled in tightly. The ski patrol guy was clearly angry with Matt and I for being out of bounds and reprimanded us as he splinted up my leg, telling us that we had lost our ski passes for the day. *Thanks dude. I just lost a limb. I think I'm all set.*

It only took a few minutes into the ride down that we found out why the run was closed. We had to cross a bubbling ravine and as I was tugged across it in the red sled behind the snowmobile, Matt had to take off his skis, again, and wade through the mini set of rapids. Now he wasn't just sweaty from the hike, he was soaking wet in freezing Vermont and skiing down the mountain carrying my skis and poles.

He had a rough day that day. But I don't know what I would have done without him. Surely, I would not have enjoyed the view as I sat stranded in the middle of nowhere.

So here we were again, Matt and I, sitting in the waiting room of another hospital trying to make ourselves laugh. Our reminiscences of "How I Tore My ACL" became a distracting source of entertainment as we waited there together on the day of my surgery.

Finally, I was called in. "Webster? Webster. We are ready for you," said a nurse standing in the waiting room in full scrubs. "Come with me, sweetheart. We are going to get prepped."

Matt and I got up to go in together, but she motioned for him to stay behind in the waiting room. "Patients only, honey," she said. "We will come get you when she's finished."

I was not prepared to be separated so abruptly, so this threw me into a new level of anxiety. *I need him with me!*

Matt gave me a hug, told me he loved me and that I would be fine, and promised he would see me soon.

Okay. Here we go. Deep breath. One, two, three, push. Crossing through the double-wide hospital doors between the waiting room and the surgical suite was like crossing into another universe. Despite the whole ACL blip the year before, I was new to the business of surgery. The whole thing amazed and confounded me.

I was put into the typical exhibitionist backless gown that doesn't close all the way, and adorned with a hair net and a pair of booties. After multiple rounds of interviews in which I repeatedly recited my name, age, and date of birth, I got marked up with a Sharpie pen so the doctor "wouldn't miss."

I would be having a lymph node removed from the right side of my neck to get biopsied. They would take this peanut-sized mound out of my neck, slice it in half, and evaluate it under a microscope right there in the surgery room.

That was the moment I was waiting for.

The whole time I was getting interviewed and drawn on, my mind was running wild. *I wonder how many mistakes they had to make to install this level of checks and balances? What happens if they make a mistake with me? What if they mistakenly switch the tissue samples and give me the wrong diagnosis? What IS the wrong diagnosis? Would that be "You have*

cancer," or would that be "Everything looks normal,
good luck to you"? Which would be worse?

*Oh my god, I'm here getting a cancer biopsy. What
if it really is cancer? Then what happens? Am I going
to die? How many years would I have? How did I even
get here!? What did I do wrong!? But then again, shit
happens, right!? I will just deal with it, right?! Fehking
shit.*

Once prepped, I got wheeled around in a rolling cot
in the gown, booties, and hair net, while everyone else
was walking the halls fully dressed. The wheeled ride,
though energy efficient, made me feel even more sickly
and pathetic in the hospital. And it seemed that each
person with a clipboard that I was wheeled past had
me confirm again who I was. These small stops in the
halls seemed random to me, and they were always
with a new, fully sterilized person in headgear and
goggles, so it was almost like a pop quiz to confirm I
was still me, that I hadn't been swapped out with
some imposter. In my case, I was feeling a little like
the latter as I was wheeled in to the meat locker that
was the surgery room.

It only took the ACL reconstruction, one wisdom
tooth removal back in college, and an ovarian cyst to
make anesthesiologists my favorite people. I had
learned quickly that those guys are always my best
friends. Julie, Trevor, Anna. I remember them all. No
matter how dozed, dazed, or dopey I am, theirs are

the names I call when I feel any sort of pinch, prod, or poke. Or even if I feel awake at all, really, let's be honest.

Because of my high levels of adrenaline, a fast metabolism, and my constant asking for more, I always get the same amount of drugs you would give a small horse. I've been told I have a habit of calling out to the anesthesiologists quite often, mid procedure. For instance, I demanded from Julie another "hit of the good stuff" during the removal of my wisdom teeth. That was the time that I ended up sliding off the sloping dentist's chair when we finished, having been substantially overserved.

With the ACL, it was Trevor who couldn't believe I was still coherent after giving me the double dose. "Please sir, may I have some more?" I apparently asked.

And it was Anna who let me stay hooked up to the morphine drip for an extra twenty minutes as we waited for my ovarian cyst to shrink because I was having a good dream. *Thanks, Anna.*

All this begging, and it turns out I actually get quite nauseous when I wake up from these drug-induced benders. Anesthesia tends to turn on me, that volatile goddess of a drug. So, why does unconscious me do this to herself? Who knows. But there we were, Anesthesia and I, about to meet again.

As I got airlifted onto the cold steel table like they would do if all my limbs were falling off, Nadine leaned over me and introduced herself. She said she would be "taking care of me today." *Ahhhh.* I knew what that meant. "Hi, Nadine," I said with my sweetest smile. "Just so you know, I have a very fast metabolism. Faster than the average bear."

I knew this was code for "I metabolize anesthesia quickly, so please keep the refills acomin'." She smiled and told me not to worry.

"We will just make sure you are nice and relaxed then," she said soothingly as she hooked me up to the relaxant. *Oh, happiness.*

Despite the surgery room being cold, sterile, and white, there was music playing. Lynyrd Skynyrd pulsed through the room. Soon the doctors and nurses began to look like little Oompa-Loompas in their blue-scrub onesies, masked faces, and white gloved hands. They shuffled happily and methodically around the room, nodding to each other and pulling this lever or pressing that button. The only part of their faces that was visible was their eyes, and I tried to distinguish one from the other as each approached the table by gazing deep inside their souls. One lifted my arm to adjust the liquid-filled tubes to my right, another checked my pulse, another adjusted my gown to perfectly frame the Sharpie markings on my neck. "X" marked the spot. Nadine had brown eyes.

As the happy juice was drip, drip, dripping through me, I felt calm. *Whatever happens, happens. Shit happens. I'm just going to deal with it. Do what I must do. Just let it be. Whatever it is, I will figure it out. Even if I end up with some strange rare disease, I will go to Iowa to get the cure. I'm going to be fine.*

It only took a vial and a half of the relaxant to get me to surrender to this out-of-control roller-coaster of a ride. And I really leaned in to it, beginning to dare the worst. *Let's have it. I dare you. What's it going to be? An early death from cancer? Fine. A rare degenerative disease? Done. Give me whichever is worse. I'll show you how strong I am.* It was the last of my bravery rearing its head.

Then, just as the optimistic part of my brain was wildly running its steroid-pumped victory lap around my head, Dr. Surgeon swung open the double doors. "Okay, team, we ready to get started?" he said to the room as he snapped on his rubber gloves. He leaned over the surgery table and asked how I was feeling.

"Great," I said with groggy enthusiasm. "We're going to be fine. I'll go to Iowa." I slurred. "We're going to fix it." I felt like we were in this together, him and I. "You're going to do great," I mumbled to him as I rolled my head over to look for Nadine.

"Okay, then. Glad you are feeling good. As we discussed earlier, this biopsy will tell us exactly what's going on," he said assuredly. "And we will look at the sample right over here." He pointed to the exorbitantly large microscope in the corner. It looked like a crouching Transformer. "You are in good hands today."

I just couldn't believe the Transformer had been in the room the whole time.

Then Nadine came over to tuck me in and send me to sleep.

"Gave you a little extra so you're nice and comfortable," she said with a wink. "Have a good sleep," she coaxed softly. And the croon of the Beatles' "Speaking words of wisdom . . ." faded away as I drifted weightlessly into the black.

Like no time had passed, I groggily "woke up" to the spin of the wheeled bed rounding a corner. The fluorescent lights swirled above me. Dr. Surgeon was leaning over the side of the railing, and keeping up with the blurring speed of the bed. "It's Hodgkin lymphoma," he said with energetic definition, in the way that people on Jeopardy declare the winning answer. I tried to process these words by staring at his mouth and repeating his lip movements.

My grogginess dulled my senses and his level of energy deeply confused me. *Was that the right or wrong diagnosis? I can't remember which one was worse. He sounds like he said the right one, but . . . what did he say again?*

Then words flooded my head. *Hodgkin lymphoma. Cancer. Lymphoma. Cancer. Cancer of the blood. Lymphatic. Systemic. Small cell, B-cell, T-cell. Shit.* The daring bravery that I had valiantly dozed off with was gone. Nowhere in sight.

Is it really cancer? How do I feel right now? Am I relieved? No. No, I'm fehking not. How many years do I have left? What do I do now? Why is Dr. Surgeon so happy? Shit. It's over. Where's Nadine?? Where's Matt?? Is this real?! Am I going to die?! Since my motor skills were still turned off, the questions ran frantic laps in my head, swirling themselves into a pile up. I was going to be sick.

The next thing I remember was sitting propped up in the recovery room sipping an apple juice box with a curved puke tray on my lap. I could hear the buzz of the halls, the clicks of heels, and the rhythmic beeps of machines. There was no music in the recovery room. No more Oompa-Loompas. The soft blue curtains hung at each side of my bed, hiding me from my beeping neighbors. I was positioned perpendicular to the hall and a large clock ticked and tocked on the wall in front of me. Six o'clock, it said. I stared ahead and took another sip out of the miniature, child-sized straw. Trying to sort out reality from the imaginary while all hopped up on anesthesia is like trying to solve a Rubik's Cube with boxing gloves on.

How long have I been in here? It can't have been three hours. Where is Matt? Where is the doctor? Did Hodgkin lymphoma happen? Is it over? Then, throb, throb, throb went my neck. Piercing pain shot out of my collarbone, up into my head and down my arm. I sat paralyzed with the juice box now crushed in my hand. I raised my other arm to touch the incision, but the needle that was taped to the top of my hand jutted out of place and a different jolt of pain seized that arm. I tried to call out, but no noise came out. The swelling had taken away my voice and my birdlike chirps went unheard in the busy halls. Immobile, mute, and in insurmountable amounts of pain, the walls started to close around me.

Someone help me. I have cancer. I'm probably going to drop dead any minute! I need help RIGHT NOW. Nadine! Where are you?! How can I get a nurse in here? Someone come help me! Where are these people? They drop a bomb like that and then disappear?! What kind of establishment is this?!

And then it dawned on me. The only thing I could think to do was to launch my juice box into the hallway. *That'll get 'em.* And like launching a hand grenade from a bunker, I chucked my empty, crumpled-up juice box out into the hall with the arm that wasn't connected to the machine.

After the first box, no one came. *I need more ammo.* I looked to my left and found two more juice boxes on the table next to me. I lobbed those out into the hall one after the next, and because they were full ones, they hit the hard, glossy floor with much more of a satisfying thud before they splattered their guts out in front of me.

Just as I was about to throw the puke bucket out into the hall, a nurse hurriedly rounded the turn into my sheeted bunker. I was sorry to have missed watching the puke tray splatter the floor, but then I was quickly reminded of the piercing, throbbing pain engulfing my upper body.

"I'm here, I'm here," she said out of breath. "I just went to get you some more pain meds and it looks like you woke up. Just my luck, I've been sitting with you for hours!" She was calm and attentive as she refilled my drip.

Even though I reluctantly realized that I had misjudged the situation, I refused to part with my scowl. "May I please have another juice box?" I asked, regretting I had forfeited all of mine.

"Yes, sweetheart," she said as she knelt on her hands and knees to wipe up the yellow puddles on the floor. "Now that you're up, I'll go get your boyfriend, okay?"

"Thanks," I said sheepishly. Her niceness was taking the wind out of my tantrum.

Drip, drip, drip went the machine. I watched the serum glide through the clear plastic into the vein on the back of my hand.

What am I going to do? How does this start? How will it end? I'm scared. What will this will do to me? How will this change me? I have forfeited the reigns on this. I don't have control over this. I am at the mercy of this. I will lose myself in this. Nothing scared me more than change that was not determined on my own terms.

Back into the safety of the black I drifted, away from that bed, that hospital, and the word *lymphoma*. I wanted to disappear into that black.

When I woke up two hours later, the nurse was petting my hair and Matt sat at the end of the bed sipping his own juice box, with his hand on my leg. I could feel the sadness seep from his hand and knew the nurse had told him.

"Oh good, you're up. How are you feeling? It's been a big day for you, I know. You think you are ready to go home?" the nurse cooed.

"Uh-huh," I answered as I put two saltines in my mouth. Back in distinguishable reality, the tears now came, rising like a tide. The life that I thought I would have played out before me. It only took a one-inch incision to jolt my life off its tracks and send it careening into fiery destruction. I cried for my life lost.

Between the dry heaving and the blubbering through the saltines, Matt and I sat quietly on the bed, as the nurse went to get my clothes. I held onto my puke bucket with both hands, like a child holds her teddy bear.

"Let's get you home," Matt said. "It's been a day. Here, let me help you."

I held on to the wall next to my bed while he helped me into my pants one leg at a time. He zippered me up, put me in the wheelchair, and wheeled me out to the street corner. Still groggy and emotionally heightened, I professed my love to him the whole way out of the hospital. "I love you too, Ceece," he said.

As I sat parked on the curb and watched him hail a taxi, the cold February air stirred my senses. As his khakis skirted around Second Avenue, I thought of him and I thought of us. And I was sad.

We had only just moved in together in a beautiful, light-filled apartment. We loved going out with our friends, and we loved staying in with dinner and a movie. Sometimes we would have wild nights out as we ran from bar to bar and sometimes we would dance in the kitchen as we cooked dinner, oven mitts and all. Having always had my own place and space, it surprised me that I didn't mind his extended, endlessly long showers in the morning, the extortionately loud "breathing" at night, or how he would finish the toothpaste and leave the empty one for me to replace. We were so happy, and we were our best selves with each other. And then here I was. Here *we* were. I knew this was his fight too and I felt sad. I felt sorry. Like quicksand, the person he met was sinking into sickness.

What happens if we can't weather this? What happens if this is just too tough to watch? I would understand. Because I wouldn't be the person he met and fell in love with. Because I would become a shadow of myself. I imagined those cancer patients you see in the movies. Gray, bald, sallow, frail, and too often hopeless. I was afraid of what I would become, knowing it would be so different to who I was when we met. I was afraid of losing love, as I changed forms right there on the curb outside of the hospital.

When we got home that night, Matt tucked me in bed, brought me tea and soup, and lay next to me. He told me about all the doctors we would call tomorrow, and all the things he had learned from the research he did while he was waiting for me to wake up. That this was "curable" and that I would be "fine."

When he told me all the funny things I had said to the hospital staff, I found a little laugh somewhere down deep. "I'm scared," I whispered as we lay there. As he put his hand on mine and said, "We are going to do this together," I drifted off to sleep, back into the black.

4 THE CLOCK WITH A THOUSAND HANDS

I wish I could say that the days following my cancer diagnosis were cast in a fog, that I was stunned into paralyzed shock and urgently expedited, in a wheelchair, through to treatment by a very large and very loud nurse, ideally with road rage. That was not the case for me.

For me, the process of getting diagnosed with cancer was like running a marathon in which the finish line kept moving, so it was just out of my reach. Imagine a dog track where the dogs chase that fluffy, little bunny lap after lap. I was the dog out in front, the one clenching its medical records as the pages flapped in the wind.

After Dr. Surgeon diagnosed me in the hospital, he simply said that he was happy to give me a recommendation for an oncologist, "That is, unless you want to find your own doctor, which patients usually prefer to do." *Find my doctor? I did already. I found you!* His buck stopped there, basically.

Like getting dropped off on the first day of school at a new school, I felt abandoned and alone. And rather than being swept off to receive urgent treatment after finally getting to an official diagnosis of cancer, I had no idea what to do next. Even worse, I was haunted by the thought that I could croak at any moment.

The morning after surgery, I woke up with a throbbing pain in my neck and a relentless headache. I only opened one eye in hopes that it had all been a dream. The Oompa-Loompas, Nadine, the juice box grenades—perhaps I had imagined it all. *Nope. That really happened.*

I sat up in bed and reached for my laptop to get some answers. Matt had gone to work, and I was alone. My room was bright and sunny. It was oddly quiet for being within earshot of Sixth Avenue. *So now what? What do I do now?* I wondered.

Words, statistics, and facts filled the room, coming at me like a tennis ball machine had gone rogue: *Nine thousand cases diagnosed per year. A 65–85 percent survival rate. Advanced stage. Early stage. More male than female. Age 20–35. Blood cancer. Bone marrow. Tests positive for Epstein-Barr virus. Cause unknown. Hodgkin versus Non-Hodgkin. Reed Sternberg cells. Uncommon types. Rare types. Tumors. Lymphocytes. Normal cells. Abnormal cells. Fast progression. Slow progression. Bone marrow biopsy. Erythrocyte sedimentation. Nodular sclerosis. Newly diagnosed. Relapsed. Refractory. Reoccurrence. Hematologist. Radiation oncologist. Second opinions. Third opinions. Treatment decisions. Chemotherapy. Immunotherapy. Radiation. High dose. Prolonged. Stem cell transplantation. Fertility defects. Remission rate. Survival rate. Holy shit. Survival rates vary patient to patient. Treatments vary patient to patient. Depends on stage and type of Hodgkin's. Stage and type. Live or die? Stage and type.* Even as I was being bombarded with information, I found little to no definitive answers. Stages I through IV seemed to range from a sneeze to a five-year survival rate.

The last description I read ended with a recommendation to "work with your doctor to get a personalized treatment plan based on your lymphoma's specific stage and type." The very thought of this exhausted me. Nothing in my life had prepared me for this. *I don't have a doctor yet. I have no idea what stage or type I am. I have no idea what is growing in me, how long I have, or how fast it is spreading as I*

*sit here in bed! All I know is that I have Hodgkin
lymphoma, isn't that enough?*

I shut my laptop and raised my tired body from
my soft white sheets. As I passed the window in front
of me, I paused to stare blankly at the skyline that
sprawled out in front of me. I watched the pigeons
swish and swoop across the sky. *I wish I was them.*

Then I called my parents. *They'll know what to do
next.*

"It's official, people. I'm *probably* going to live, but
there could be a forty percent chance I am dying. I
might have thirty more years in me, or I could have
just five. I might just need to take a pill, but I could
also need a stem cell transplant and copious amounts
of radiation on top of chemo. Which might work, but
maybe not."

"Okay. Get off Google. That's not going to help
anything." My father was always the practical one in
dramatic situations. Hearing this reminded me of the
time he told me to get down from the tree in the front
yard when I had perched myself fifty feet up on a
spindly branch that was precariously swaying in the
wind.

"First things first. We need a good doctor," my
mother said with assertion from the background. She
then grabbed the phone and rattled off a list of her
friends that we could call to get their doctor

recommendations. It was amazing how many cancer people my parents knew.

This was the same strategy that Matt was taking as he was pretending to do work in his office in midtown. Basically, he, my mother, and I were calling every cancer friend we had. People who'd had cancer or whose relatives had cancer, or who worked in a health-related profession and had good contacts. By mid-afternoon, I had a laundry list of potential doctors in hand.

Being in New York, I knew I had access to the best medical care in the country, if not the best cancer care in the world: Memorial Sloan-Kettering, New York-Presbyterian/Weill Cornell Medical Center, NYU Langone Medical Center, Mount Sinai Beth Israel Hospital. *How hard can it be? Call the hospital, go in, get treatment. Bing, bang, boom. Lymphoma OVER. Shit happened, and I'm just going to deal with it, right?*

"Hi, I have just been diagnosed with Hodgkin lymphoma." The words sounded so foreign to me as they came out of my mouth. "I would like to see if I can get an appointment to see Dr. Board of Lymphoma Research Foundation, Dr. Awarded Member of the Society of Clinical Investigation, or Dr. Leadership Committee of Hematology Subspecialty. Do they have any availabilities?" I asked, my voice only slightly shaking.

"Let me transfer you to each of their admins. Please hold," the receptionist said mechanically. Three hours later, I had memorized the words to the hold music, spoken with six physician's assistants, sent my records twice, and was now on two percent phone battery so was demoted to the floor of my apartment, deflated, and crumpled up next to the plug. I had crossed off half the names on my list. The next available appointment for any of them was two months away. According to my research, two months was a bit of a gamble. I hesitated as I couldn't believe what was about to come out of my mouth.

"Yeah . . . Well, I don't think that I can wait two months," I said to the last assistant, shocked by my own seriousness. "Is there anything you can do?" She apologized and promised she'd call me if anything opened up. I took that to mean that someone needed to die before I could get in to see the doctor whose front desk she staffed.

Gruesome, but I began to think of how I could knock someone off that list. *Unplug their IV? Push their wheelchair down the stairs? It wouldn't take much, since they are cancer patients probably on the threshold of death's door anyway. AH! Wait. I'm a cancer patient! Fehking hell.*

Matt, my mother, and I spent three days on the phone with hospitals trying to get me in. Each assistant and front desk operator had the same robotic response, which I struggled to comprehend. *Why aren't you hearing me?! I could be dying! I might not be around on July 10th at 2:30 PM if you don't put me on the schedule NOW! It's February, for Christ's sake!*

Then my mental tension would build. *Thinking of Christ, I should probably start going to church, just in case. We don't even know what stage I am, or what type of Hodgkin I have! It could be the WORST KIND! It could be classic Hodgkin or Nodular Lymphocyte-Predominant Hodgkin, in which case we are REALLY in trouble. I could have one of the rare kinds, or the rapidly progressing one! You don't know! Get me in NOW!*

At a time when I felt like I should be the center of the receptionists' concern, my panic wasn't getting the response that it demanded. Of course, I had not realized that they get basically the same call day in and day out from dozens of people. These people were numb to the sound a world makes when it comes crashing down. They were not strangers to the high-pitched tone of desperation that prospective patients employ or the throaty gurgle of a plea. My case was no different. Get in line.

Over the next seventy-two hours, the days on the phone demanded relentless persistence and patience, which was a tortuous combination for me. To me, the repetitive calls met with the lack of urgency on the other end were driving me even further into a fanatic frenzy, which spun itself into a unique brand of a devil-may-care hysteria. I would call offices again and again, speaking to the same poor woman call after call, asking if anyone had died yet. Considering the definition of insanity is to do the same thing over and over while expecting a different result, I was holding a one-way ticket to Crazy Town.

All the while, I just wanted to stop and allow myself to *be* sick. I had finally gotten a diagnosis and I was desperate to be done, to rest. Exhaustion had driven me to find a doctor. Now I was ready to just collapse into sickness and further fatigued by following through. Just shut my eyes and give in. But I couldn't. I had to keep up. I was almost there, right? *One more call. One more minute on hold. One more faxed medical release form. One more day. One more.* I had to keep running, all the while fearing the worst. It was a heart pounding, anxiety-propelling, unsympathetic marathon of a job to get myself to treatment.

"Anything yet?" I would ask Matt as I crawled in to bed at the end of the day.

"No, not yet. But we'll get there," he said assuredly. "I'm calling more offices tomorrow. I don't want you to worry. We will get in."

My symptoms were in full throttle at this point, and I would tuck myself into bed with sweaters and socks on, a heating pad, and a truckload of Tylenol

PM. The aches would wake me up at three AM like clockwork, and I would raise my pounding body from my warm, sweaty spot on the bed to get into the shower. I would rock back and forth, back and forth. Most times, I would cry, letting the warm water blend with my tears. *I don't have two months. Why don't they hear me? Why won't anyone take me? Just take me.* All I wanted to do was rest, to sleep, to disappear, to go back to the black.

Then, on the fourth day of phone calls, and by some miracle on Thirty-Fourth Street, Matt got a lead. Through the webbed network that is New York, we found an "in" through Matt's father's friend's daughter's doctor. At this point, we weren't just pulling strings, we were grabbing at maritime ropes trying to get into one of the top cancer centers.

Matt's family's connection was at Weill Cornell in the Hematology and Medical Oncology center. Weill Cornell's lymphoma program was widely recognized, and this oncologist was one of the best in the field. He was on boards, he was awarded, he was published. He specifically specialized in blood cancers, and he was the Hodgkin expert. After the connections were made, I called Dr. Hodgkin's office to make an appointment.

"Ah yes, we've been expecting your call," the office assistant said sweetly. "When would you like to come in? There is usually a three-month wait, but since you are a friend of Dr. Hodgkin, of course we are making an exception." I began to think we had pulled too hard on the ropes and someone had oversold this connection. But without batting an eye, I scheduled myself to go in the next week. No unplugging of IVs necessary. Not yet at least.

How do "normal" people do this? Do people actually WAIT the full two months? How is that possible? People must DIE waiting. Oh well, not me. I'm in. It's over. It's all going to be coasting from here.

The morning of the appointment, Matt, my mother, and I piled through the hospital's revolving door on Manhattan's Upper East Side and made our way to the Hematology/Oncology Medical Center on the third floor. My mother, who had clicked in to mother mode in the highest of gears, had flown directly in from our vacation house just for this appointment. My father, in what was ultimately an attempt to downplay the drama in all that what was happening to me, was waiting in the tropics by the phone. He was leaving all the mothering to my mother, but he couldn't resist calling me multiple times a day to check in, trying to distract me with what our dogs were doing.

"Starr Three," the receptionist in the front lobby had called the cancer center. Like a spaceship, the halls of Starr Three were bright, glossy, and sterile. Doctors and nurses in white coats flipped the pages on their clipboards as they moved swiftly down the halls. As the doctors slid through the various doors, I would catch a glimpse of a curved arm of a machine, the wheeled foot of a rolling monitor, or the frosted glass of another door leading to another corridor. The rooms beeped and clicked as we passed them. It was like seeing the inner workings of NASA. We checked in and were taken right back to meet the doctor in one of the exam rooms.

Dr. Hodgkin greeted us with firm handshakes and kind eyes. Even though he spent minimal time with conversation and formalities, he was warm and genuine, with a note of severity, which from my seat, I appreciated. We got started immediately and spent the next two hours getting the full download.

He took us through everything, from the origins of lymphoma, to side-effect management and treatment options. There we were, the three of us, huddled together on one side of the desk, nodding our heads as we listened and grappled with the situation. Throughout the appointment, Dr. Hodgkin only spoke to me. It seemed as if others were out of his focus. *Just how it should be.* When my mother asked him if what I had was Lyme's disease instead of lymphoma, he just looked at her blankly and returned to his explanation of chemotherapy treatment and toxicity levels.

After he examined me and probed around the swollen lymph nodes in my neck, chest, and groin, Dr. Hodgkin had me sit back down.

"You are in the advanced stages of Hodgkin," he said calmly and methodically. "Based on what I just felt, we are looking at Stage Three to Four. We are going to run blood and image tests to confirm, and then we move to treatment. Based on those results, we will decide on treatment type and duration. I recommend we move quickly."

Advanced stage. Stage Four. Move quickly. He must have felt tumors and bulges and all sorts of foreign things in there. Stage Four. Four. F-O-U-R. That's a forty percent chance of dying! That's a five-year life expectancy! I have no time and I need more tests! More appointments. More blood. But I'm almost there. I'm so close. Holy shit. How did this happen to me?! Oh my God. Inside I was dying of anxiety, but outwardly I kept my calm, since Dr. Hodgkin's severity deterred hysterics. "Okay," I replied, keeping my words to one syllable so as not to give away my panic.

"Once we have the blood tests and imaging results back, we can get into more detail about a treatment plan," he continued. "But for classic Hodgkin, which is the more common type of Hodgkin lymphoma, we generally treat with ABVD, which is a cocktail of four chemotherapy agents: Adriamycin, Bleomycin, Vinblastine, and Dacarbazine. It is delivered by infusion, and we will need to do a fairly rigorous schedule of every other week. Since you are in later stages, and you are young, we will hit this hard."

Cocktail of chemo. Infusion. Four separate infusions? Oh God. Rigorous. Every other week. I'm young. Too young to die. Hit this hard. How hard? Is it going to hit me hard, or just the bad, mutant cell-filled parts? Holy shit.

"Side effects drastically vary patient to patient, but nausea, considerable fatigue, skin reactions, and loss of appetite are all to be expected," said Dr. Hodgkin in the same way the weatherman predicts the weekend forecast.

"Am I going to lose my hair?" I asked with a squeak. I heard myself sound petty and vain as I asked it. What's a little hair loss when my life was at stake? The question, however, came from a different place. All the other side effects I could hide. I could tuck them behind my armor. No one needed to know. I could weather the poison of chemo. The hair though, that was going to give me away, and expose my sickness to the world. They would see me as weak, sick, broken, and changed. And that, I just couldn't handle.

"Only two thirds of patients end up losing their hair completely," Dr. Hodgkin responded.

Lose hair completely. Nausea. Severe fatigue. No appetite. I really am going to become a sick person. Everyone will know. This is really happening. Gray, sallow, frail, and broken.

Dr. Hodgkin continued speaking. "In the rare case that your lymphoma does not respond to ABVD, there is another treatment option manufactured by a German drug company. This will be our second choice as this treatment is much more toxic and we are trying to limit your exposure, as much as we can, to high toxicity levels."

"Your lymphoma," he said. My lymphoma. This is not "my lymphoma." I refuse to accept this cancer as my own! My body has turned on me! Abnormal cells. Mutant cells. I have monsters growing, dividing, and forging an army within me. They are not mine! They do not belong to me. What if the demon cells win? What if we need the Germans back up? What will it take to kill the demon cells? Whatever it is will kill the good cells too. How many cell casualties will there be? Demolished and mutated, they will lay there in the smoke. How will my body survive this? Toxic. Exposure. Radioactive. Hiroshima.

"Okay," I repeated, as I started to recognize what loomed ahead. With each explanation, chemotherapy began to etch itself out on the horizon, dark and foreboding.

"Let's talk fertility for a minute," said Dr. Hodgkin, as he took us through the implications of treatment. "Before we start the infusions, I want to give you the option to meet with a fertility specialist here at the hospital. Even though ABVD is not associated with fertility issues, the choice is yours to make and I want you to be as comfortable as possible before we start the regimen. You do have the option of freezing your eggs, *but* that will delay your first treatment by a significant amount of time. I wouldn't recommend too much of a delay, and it is my suggestion to start treatment as soon as possible. Again, the choice is absolutely up to you."

Infertility. Freeze my eggs. Don't delay treatment. Start the regimen NOW. I don't have time. I'm running out of time. But I'm twenty-nine. I'm supposed to have inconceivable amounts of time. Like I don't even THINK about time. I'm supposed to be in the height of fertility. I'm not supposed to be worrying about this. I can't believe this is happening.

I sat silent and stunned for a moment, before another wave of panic swept through my body. *What happens if I can't have children? What about Matt? Would he want to stay? Will he still love me? Choice. Choice is mine? But it's not. I don't feel like any of this is mine. I don't have a choice in any of this. Everything just keeps going and going, out of control. Out of MY control. The choice has never been mine.*

With a simple nod of my head, I agreed to see the fertility specialist the following day.

As Dr. Hodgkin patiently closed out the two-hour discussion, he reiterated that I was going to be fine. That I was in good hands. That I had the "best" kind of cancer, and I could get as close to cured as anyone with cancer can get. He reminded me that *cure* was a word not easily associated with cancer, so I was *lucky,* which was also a word not easily associated.

Best cancer. Cancer. I have cancer. Cancer is not curable. I'm broken. Hindered. Disabled. I will carry this for the rest of my life. What does the rest of my life look like? No children, no Matt, no house, no lawn. I'll be alone. I am afraid of what I will become. What if the mutant monsters win? I'd almost prefer that. I want to go back into the black. Lucky? This is not lucky. One of the nine thousand most unlucky people in the country, in fact.

With that, Dr. Hodgkin shook our hands as he told us his assistant would schedule the blood work, all staging tests, and the fertility appointment for next week. Based on the tests results, and on my decision on whether to freeze my eggs or not, the first treatment could begin as early as the week following. On a Tuesday.

As he shut the door behind him, Matt and my mother began comparing notes. I just and stared at the freezing rain that was now hitting the glass panes of the window. The clock with a thousand hands was spinning in my head. *Just one more test. One more doctor. One more day. Almost there.*

In the days that followed my appointment with Dr. Hodgkin, I ran through test after test, then I met with the fertility specialist, then had the PET CT scan in which I became radioactive and was lit up like a

Christmas tree in a scanner the size of an eighteen-wheeler.

First, I had the lung test. I was told that ABVD can impact lung function, meaning to me that the medicine could wither away my capacity to breathe. my lungs were tested to make sure that they could "withstand treatment." The test required holding my breath and then exhaling to the brink of passing out, all while sitting in a little glass box in a large room with a technician counting down from ten with their hands. *Strong enough to withstand treatment, they had said.* Treatment was sounding more and more like torture. I had no idea what was coming, but with each prod, poke and suffocating exhale into the plastic mouthpiece, the darkness on the horizon kept sending smoke signals to warn me.

Next, I met with the fertility doctor with Matt by my side.

"Well, good news. Your ovaries are very fertile and there are *plenty* of eggs," he said as he stared at the screen during my ultrasound. I lay on the table like a corn dog on a stick trying to decipher the gray and white smudges on the screen next me. *What eggs? Where are the eggs?* You may be looking at my larynx by the feel of this thing.

"Get dressed and let's chat in my office," he said as he pulled out the wand from what seemed like up inside my chest cavity.

Once in his office, he took us through our options, which didn't really sound like choices.

"If you did want to freeze your eggs, it would take four to five weeks to harvest them, and by Dr. Hodgkin's notes, that might be too long to wait. But it is up to you." *Is it up to me? If it were up to me, we wouldn't be having this conversation.*

On the one hand, I wanted to freeze my eggs because I was afraid of having my ovaries and reproductive capabilities obliterated by chemotherapy. On the other hand, I feared that perhaps those eggs in there were sick and by freezing them, I would put my unborn children at risk for some inevitable and incurable cancer. Then they would have to do what I was doing, and even though I wasn't a mother, I had bear-like instincts to protect my unborn children. Unsure of what to do, I asked the doctor what he would tell his daughter in this situation.

"Looking at your ovaries today and considering your young age, I believe you are going to be fine. Should you want to freeze your eggs, the idea would be to use them as a last resort anyway." I could tell he was uncomfortable with giving a definite response and this was the closest he could get. I looked at Matt for his opinion. He repeated, "We're going to be fine," which I knew meant, "Whatever happens, happens and I will still love you." And I felt guilty and sad for putting him in this position so early in our relationship. Despite the reassurance, I left the appointment feeling like I was walking in to a casino with my entire life savings in my hand.

And finally, the last appointment was the PET CT scan. After drinking a liter of radioactive, highlighter yellow "lemonade" with a pungent metallic after taste, I was tucked in to the enormous scanning machine. As I got motored into the beige tunnel, it was like being inside of a spaceship. As the magnets orbited my body, I imagined each of my diseased organs—the bulging lymph nodes, the infected bone marrow—all lighting up like Rudolph's nose, pulsing red. As the machine clicked its way around me, I closed my eyes and prayed. I am not a devout and pious person really. I am not a regular churchgoer, I've never confessed, and I don't know the hymns by heart. But I do talk to a God in those dire, desperate times. That day in the scanner, I prayed for me. I prayed for what I was about to endure. I prayed for the healthy cells that were left in my body. I prayed for strength. The finish line seemed right there in front of me.

It was so close, I could touch it.

5 THE BATH

On the night of my PET/CT scan, I spent the cab ride home from the hospital listening to the pessimistic side of my brain argue with the optimistic side, like two teenagers on a debate team. Its proposition was: *I bet the lymphoma has metastasized and spread throughout my entire body. I bet I lit up like the Rockefeller Center Christmas tree in there. I probably only have a week or two, tops.*

Whereupon the optimistic side countered: *No, you idiot. It can't have spread. Dr. Hodgkin said any spreading would be "incredibly rare." Next to impossible.*

Exactly. He didn't say it was impossible. It's only NEXT to impossible. Which means it could happen!

And, if you think about it, getting Hodgkin lymphoma is "incredibly rare" in the first place, so why rule this rarity out either? My odds have been shit so far. And speaking of odds, the treatment might not work anyway.

Yes, it will. It will work! He said it will work!

I'll end up dying a horrible, painful, suffocating death in a matter of months if not weeks.

No, I won't. I'm not going to die. He said I won't die.

Okay then, I'll live forever. But I'll be covered in tumors, most of my organs will need to be cut out, and then I'll have a few amputations done. I'll die alone as a stumpy, lumpy, deformed shell of a person, who can't even have cats because she doesn't have any hands to open a can of tuna. Won't that be nice?

Sixty-seven hours and two sleepless nights later, Dr. Hodgkin called with the results of the scan. I heard the phone ring and reached my hand out from the sofa where I was lying in my pajamas with my slippered feet up the wall. "Everything came out as we predicted," the doctor said calmly. I swung my feet around and sat up, my inner optimist wanting to be upright to hear the news.

He continued, "We are going to go ahead and move forward with our treatment plan as discussed, but due to the progression of the lymphoma we saw, we are going to run a rigorous course of ABVD, which means that we are going to treat you with twelve infusions, and we will start in five days."

Shit, I thought as I brought my fuzzy sheepskin slippers to the floor and sat on the edge of the sofa. Aloud I said, "Okay. Tuesday. Great." Then, trying to steer the answer in my favor, I asked, "And just to confirm, you didn't see any metastases on the scan, right? No abnormal growths or large tumors?"

"No, we did not. Everything came out as we predicted," he repeated.

"And chemo is going to work? I am going to live?"

"Most likely."

Most likely? Somehow that wasn't entirely reassuring. After I hung up, I found myself standing in the middle of my living room holding my phone with a sweaty hand. Everything was blank. I didn't know what to feel, or how to feel it. I felt like I was numbingly putting one foot in front of the other, powerless and out of control. The floor seemed to sway beneath me. This was real, and it was all happening. I called my parents, who spoke words of encouragement that just bounced right to the floor in front of me. I couldn't hear any of it, except the "I love yous" at the end, before we hung up.

I shuffled over to the living room window of my apartment and looked out toward the West. It was the early evening and the sky had already begun to turn pink and orange. Winter days were so short. The large glass windows radiated the February cold, and my bones were starting to ache. I set down the phone and decided to draw a bath.

As I heated the water, my mind went to the comfort of a checklist in my head. Like a pacifier, I sucked and chewed on the preparation plans for Tuesday. I just couldn't wait to strike a satisfying X through a series of imaginary boxes, one by one. *All the doctor's appointments are done—I can cross those off. No more biopsies, no more phone calls, no more tests or scans. Diagnostic phase done.* Check. *Treatment starting next week. Tuesday ten AM. Need to call Human Resources and get set up on disability. Add that. And then I need to pick up those prescriptions that Dr. Hodgkin called in. Add that too.*

I took off my pajamas in the bathroom and looked at the body in the mirror. I was thin and frail. My collarbones protruded and cast a shadow on my chest, which made my skin look thin and bruised. *What is happening?* I lowered my aching body into the warm, still water, leaned back on a rolled-up towel I had put behind my neck, and closed my eyes, wondering, *Is this how old people feel?* That would be something to look forward to. Living to be old.

I felt surprisingly calm in the silence of my apartment. I could hear the distant hum of the traffic going up Sixth Avenue and the periodic shuffling of ice cubes from the freezer in the kitchen. I could hear my breath and the drip, drip, drip of the faucet. As I sat in stillness under the weight of the water, my thoughts drifted to my impending treatment.

Why doesn't anyone ever want to say the word chemotherapy? *They avoid it like it's a bad word. They want to make sure that my body 'can handle it'. Rigorous, they said. Hit it hard, they said. It will help me, they said. We'll give you support, they said. Toxic. Damage to lung tissue. Heart problems. Kidney problems. Nerve damage. Infertility. Risk of second cancer. Early menopause. Kidney and urinary problems. Cognitive problems. Difficulty focusing. Memory loss. Chemo. Fehk.*

There was nothing I could do other than to wait for chemotherapy to slam into me and sweep me up in its violent wake.

In the calm of the bath, I found myself turning inward and speaking to my body as if it were a neglected child. It didn't even know what was coming. The towel cradled my neck as I stared at my toes. *Be still, body. We made it, body. We can fall into sickness now, body. I'm here, body.* I could feel the pulse, pulse, pulse. *Here we go, body. Brace yourself, body. Stay with me, body. I'm going to take care of you, body. Be strong, body. I'm sorry, body. Warmth and weight. Wait. Pulse pulse pulse.*

As I watched my stomach rise and fall, rise and fall with each of my breaths, I thought about my stomach, my toes, my hands, my arms, my elbows, my legs. And I felt sad for them. I felt sorry. I had forgotten my body, neglected it, silenced it, and ignored it for most of my life. Because I was twenty-nine, of course I believed there always would be a tomorrow. But now this body was broken. *I was selfish, body. I forgot about you, body. I did this to you, body. I'm sorry, body.*

I trembled at the very thought of receiving twelve infusions of chemotherapy. *Was my behavior responsible for inviting cancer in?* My workweeks had been laden with deadlines, and the stress of proving myself, of needing to belong and please everyone around me. I would skip lunches, not drink enough water, and disregard the clock at night as I worked against that last deadline, ignoring how tired I was. Even after working late nights, I would wake up and go to an early morning spin class or do ninety minutes of Bikram yoga despite my occasional snore during Savasana.

Weekends were usually full of dinners, dancing, and long brunches. And when my friends and I would run from bar to bar on a Saturday, we would order more beer, say, "Let's get Buffalo wings," and I would forget about those blisters from the night before. After a few drinks, I would forget that my tongue was dry and my muscles sore, and that I was tired, because I was so busy with the life I was leading.

No stopping. Never stopping. I felt that I always had to keep going. Chasing what was next.

Watching my stomach rise and fall with my breath as I sat in the tub was like feeling around for a numb lower lip after you leave the dentist's office. My body felt so foreign to me, that I became aware of it. Slowly, I started to listen to it, and trying to decode its foreign language that I didn't know how to speak.

But I felt it. I felt my body fighting that day in the bath. My body was brave, and I was not. It was fighting blindly and viciously, while I Googled potential side effects, feared the repercussions of not freezing my eggs, and preempted total, collateral disaster.

As I got ready for bed that night, I took extra time brushing my teeth, smoothed cream slowly and methodically over my face and hands, and searched my medicine cabinet for a multivitamin. I felt pathetic about my meager attempts to take care of myself, but it was the only way I knew how to say thank you, how to be kind, how to say that I'm going to do this better. *I am with you, body.*

I drew up the next day's checklist in my head as I fell asleep that night. *Take out laundry and dry cleaning. Cancel all remaining class packages: Spin Cycle. High-Intensity Training. Yoga. Get paper towels and toilet paper. Put "out of office" message on. Find loungewear that doesn't make me look like a sick person. Maybe house slippers? Change the sheets. Get milk.* And I drifted off to sleep as I counted my breaths.

6 LIMBOLAND

After my deep, Ambien-infused sleep, I woke up with renewed energy. Since my symptoms didn't wake up until mid-afternoon, the mornings were when I felt the best. With a few short hours of feeling like myself, I had gotten in to the habit of cramming a full day into that five-hour time slot and getting as much done as I could before the day depleted my batteries and I was left achy, pale, and tired. Physically, my days resembled the evolution of mankind, but backward, as I went from sturdily upright in the morning to scraping my knuckles on the floor by 3 PM.

At 10 AM that day, with my batteries fully charged and my engine revved, I put the list I had drawn up in my head the night before to paper and prepared to tick the items off one by satisfying one. *Vroom, vroom.*

First on the list was to call Human Resources at the agency to give them the update on the final diagnosis and treatment plan. "Yeah. I know. Can you believe it? Crazy," I said to my HR manager on the phone. "Yes, I'll be doing chemo. . . . Of course, I'm coming back! It'll just be six months. . . . Thank you, but it'll be totally fine!" I was clearly in denial. Just a short ten minutes later, I was registered under disability and had put my out of office on.

First thing, done. I drew a thick line with a Sharpie over the line item at the top of my list and smiled to myself, remembering how great it felt to cross shit off. Sometimes at work, I would make a list of already completed to-dos, just so I could cross them out.

Off to a roaring start, I then called my parents to check in before I hit the streets. "I'm headed out shortly to get shit done," I said to them. I read off my list to show off my productivity.

"Okay, but don't tire yourself out. It's important that you rest, and that sounds like a lot for one day," my mother said with caution.

"Oh, stop it, Carolyn, she's not on her death bed," I heard my father say from the other room. "It's a few errands. Jesus."

"I know, I know, Mum. I'll be done before I get tired," I replied, brushing off her concern like I was swatting away a pesky fly. I was on my father's side here and I thought I could run against the clock.

I experienced three distinct emotions during the Limboland that was my pre-chemo nesting period.

Awareness. I became supremely aware of the impending differences that I would have from the rest of the world around me, as a sick person. In anticipation, I started to mark the comparisons and then separate myself from the world.

Anger. I became profoundly angry that cancer was happening to me.

Conformity. Despite the impending differences that were hurdling my way, I was desperate to hold on to my normal self for as long as I could. I was desperate to fit in, keep who I wanted to be alive, and hold my place and my plan intact, with the same intensity that someone has when clinging to the edge of a very, very, *very* high cliff.

Awareness

Invigorated by my morning's mission, I sprung out the door and into my Chelsea neighborhood to tackle the rest of my list with focused determination. *Okay. What's first? Loungewear. I need loungewear. And then the workout packages. Need to cancel those. Last will be the drug store to pick up those prescriptions that Dr. Hodgkin called in. Be home by three PM. That gives me four hours and thirty-seven minutes.*

Like a stealth arctic Eskimo, I made my way through the New York City tundra swathed in my entire winter closet, hat ears aflappin'. As I made my way over to Fifth Avenue, I bounced my bundled body over sheets of ice, snow mounds, and soggy garbage. My head poked out of my tightly bound scarf like a turtle from its shell, but because the February air was biting my cheeks, I only starting sweating through my first layer of coats by the time I made it to the corner.

Rather than seal pelts and whale blubber, my first hunt was for loungewear: soft, stretchy pajama bottoms, cozy oversized sweatshirts, and luxuriously comfy socks. I scurried over the icy sidewalk trying to cover as much ground as quickly as I could. Like the White Rabbit in *Alice in Wonderland,* I kept checking the time, and with each passing minute, I'd be startled into a new, higher gear. *Four hours and twenty-six minutes. Energy at ninety-five percent. I have to hurry. I have to get everything I need. I have to beat the ache. So, I'll be ready. Ready for Tuesday.*

Because I was preparing for apocalyptic sickness, I thought it safe to assume that I would be wearing a lot of pajamas. Three seasons worth of pajamas. I would be wearing so many pajamas throughout the six months of therapy, that I would need an assortment to match the season, the temperature, the time of day, my mood, and whether I was having visitors. When I did the math, that was a lot of loungewear.

In the first department store, I went straight for the "sleep wear" floor. It was the first time that I realized that the "sleepwear" department is only ten percent full of actual pajamas and ninety percent full of bolstering, squeezing, and stringy things that are definitely not meant for sleeping.

As I got to the top of the escalator and saw the clock on the wall, I lurched into a higher speed. *Have to hurry! Have to get shit done!* I dodged passed the masked and corseted mannequins and through the aisles of girdles to reach the droopy rack in the far back corner of the store. *Jesus. This is it?! What a sad display.* My fingers fluttered over padded pink bath robes with stray gray hairs stuck to the sleeves, and sagging floor-length cotton night shifts layered with eyelet frills. The dressing gowns had extra-large buttons for arthritic fingers and there was a bucket full of bedroom slippers that looked like moon boots made of duvet covers. The moon boots were a large one-size-fits-all that provided ample room for bulging bunions and long spindly toes. This tiny section in the back of the store was clearly for the over eighties, but I grabbed a floral muu muu anyway and tried it on.

Once draped in the yards of flowery polyester, I stared at myself in the mirror as I raised my arms so the fabric under them looked like the wings of a flying squirrel. *It's not so bad. I can pull this off. If I twirl just right, it kind of looks like an evening gown.* I imagined myself twirling around my apartment like a top. *I'll take it. Let's keep moving.* I checked the clock. *How did that take thirty minutes?! Eek! Have to hurry!*

I dashed and darted my back through the rows of lacey underpinnings and wiry push-up bras to check out. Just as I was about to pull in to the checkout line, a very tall and slender woman casually swept in in front of me. *Ugh. Damnit.* Her legs were twice the length of mine and perched on top of them was waif-like and thin with freckle-less skin full to the brim with collagen. She must have been a model and she was gorgeous. While I was giving her tight and perky backside the evil eye for cutting me off, I became profoundly aware of my own body. For anyone who has ever stood next to, or in this case behind, a model, you know what that feels like. Every insecurity you have about your physical appearance comes screaming out. Throw cancer into the mix, and you are toast. To me, I was standing next to beauty and youth right before I was about to lose mine. She was holding the lacey lingerie that I used to buy, and I was holding an enormous heap of floral fabric preparing for apocalyptic sickness. Her skin was flawless and mine seemed now had raised, purple scars.

I looked around to watch the other customers on the open floor as they made their way through the sections. A woman was buying an evening gown, and I became starkly aware that I wasn't going to be going to any parties. Another had an armful of active wear, and I knew that I was on my way to cancel my class packages. And now, this freak of nature model stood in front me holding tiny pieces of lace and silk, and I became staunchly aware of how "unsexy" I was about to become. Looking around the store, I became intensely aware of how cancer was already starting to overhaul my carefully designed. Everything was starting to change, and it was spinning out my control.

While the model took a long-legged stride up to the register in front of me, I tried to rewrite the script and imagine my life in my new muu muu. *I'll be like the grand dame of Twenty-First Street, taking visitors and serving nice cheese. I'll be reclined on my chaise longue with my floral muu muu spread out like a fan around me. I'll wear big, dangly earrings—hell I'll wear all of my jewelry at once. Maybe I'll even get a turban when the hair goes. My life will be loungy and reclining. Yes, that's it. Loungy and reclining.*

When I reached the till, "Susan" the clerk greeted me and reached for my crumpled ball of florals.

"Would you like it gift wrapped?" she asked with a cheerful smile, obviously thinking it was for someone else.

"No thanks, it's just for me," I said as I spent extra time digging through my bag for my wallet to avoid eye contact. My eyes had welled with tears, and I didn't want her to see them.

Anger

I collected the bag, wiped my eyes, and headed out of the store. I was eager to pitch myself back into high speed as I passed the clock at the top of the escalator. *No time for tears. Three hours and thirty-nine minutes left. Battery at seventy percent. Have to hurry.* Still needing more sets of loungewear, I bolted down Fifth Ave, darting from store to store, checking the time as I whirled through the glass door vestibules. It was as if each swing of the stores' double doors pushed me faster and faster as I ran against the clock.

Four stores later, I was laden with multiple bags filled with yoga pants, sweatshirts, socks, and muu muus, which I had started calling "lounge gowns" to the confusion of store clerks. Even the weight of the bags couldn't slow my speed as I hopped and slid my way back to my apartment to drop off the first load. After piling the bags in the lobby, I rung out my arms after their weight had cut off the circulation to my hands. I fumbled for my phone to check the time. *Two hours and eleven minutes left. Battery at fifty percent.*

As I went back out onto the street, I tried to talk myself into finishing my list with some level of tactful normalcy, and not winding myself up into obsessive compulsive craziness. Basically, I tried to tell myself to calm the *fehk* down. Feeling like I was holding back a four-hundred horsepower Maserati, I tried to walk slowly and methodically the two blocks back to Fifth Avenue. I tried to focus on things like my breath and the feeling of my feet in my boots, instead of the passing minutes. I found proof that my focused effort on taking deep breaths was working when I started choking on massive gulps of freezing air. Just as I closed my eyes to look for my inner chi (wherever the hell that was), an enormous shoulder slammed in to me, and like a small bumper car hitting the tire of an eighteen-wheeler, I bounced off the arm and the curb, into the urine-spackled snow plow mound on the corner of Twenty-First Street.

"Watch where you're going!" the man yelled over his shoulder as I lay sprawled out in the snow.

As I got up from my full body imprint in the dirty mound, a gnarled ball of snow and garbage got in my boot and slithered down to melt on the exposed skin between my sock and my pant leg. This, my ultimate torture, threw me over the edge and into a deep pit of curdling rage. The dirty sludge on my coat and now in my boot launched me into a maddened anger and I frantically vaulted and heaved myself around the sidewalk, violently shaking my legs and arms. To the other people on the street, I must have looked like I was worshipping some kind of burial ground as I leapt, shook, and flailed around.

And then the rage took over. The screws had shaken themselves lose and the wheels had flown off the wagon. Like the time I got food poisoning in Mexico, the anger ruptured out in a vile, toxic mess. *I JUST GOT DIAGNOSED WITH FEHKING CANCER. WATCH WHERE I'M GOING!? I'M GOING TO FEHKING CHEMO NEXT WEEK! WHAT THE FEHK IS WRONG IS WITH YOU?!*

I was angry at the guy with the behemoth shoulders for not knowing that I was sick. I was angry at everyone who was looking at me on the street. I felt like somehow, people should automatically and telepathically know that I needed extra space in the crowd, that I should cross the street first, that my order should be before theirs, that I didn't have to wait in line, that I had the right of way. I stood planted in the middle of sidewalk as I tried to scrape off the toxic smell of the rancid garbage from my coat, squealing with each swipe.

Even though the dirt and sewage water were off me, the internal rage was more of a crimson stain.

Like the Queen of Hearts when she was disobeyed, my face was now the scarlet shade of maniacal anger and I heatedly trudged the rest of the way to Fifth Avenue. I stomped a straight and unforgiving line to the next item on my list, brushing aside pets and small children. *MOVE OUT THE WAY OR OFF WITH YOUR HEAD!*

Conformity

My sweaty palms left fog marks on my phone as I checked the time. *One hour and forty-nine minutes left. Battery at thirty percent.* I huffed and puffed my way in to the spin studio around the corner.

This was the first workout package I needed to cancel since I had ten classes left in my account, and for those who are familiar with New York City fitness classes, that is the equivalent of owning a designer handbag. A big one made of a very rare leather with lots of hardware and several compartments.

I was cancelling my packages because strenuous workout classes did not fit my understanding of cancer and chemo. I wasn't sure how the therapy would affect me, but when I imagined a typical chemo patient, they sure as shit weren't sweating on a bike, tapping it back and forth while dancing to techno remixes. They certainly weren't bopping their bald heads to the beat of Today's Top Hits while turning up the torque. They weren't crab crawling across the floor of early morning HIT classes, and they weren't boiling their bodies with ninety minutes of profuse sweating in Bikram yoga.

As I passed through the shiny glass doors of the studio, I was met with a blast of warm sweaty air and the pulsing beat of Justin Timberlake's claimed inability to "stop the feeling . . ."

From the look of the room, I could tell that a class had just finished, and another was about to start. The check-in area at the front felt charged with energy and swarmed with bouncy blonds clad in neon sports bras who were hurriedly grabbing at pairs of shoes and water bottles from the girls at reception. The receptionists behind the counter swiftly ricocheted between checking people in at the counter and reaching for the wall of rent-a-shoes. They seemed to be-bop around behind the desk, exalting the regulars with hugs and hellos, and sending them on their way with a "Go be your best *you*, girl!" or "Believe in yourself!" and "Keep pushing those boundaries, Kelly!"

To say I felt out of place on that particular day would be an understatement. I felt like a bowling ball standing next to a bunch of sparkly, neon pins. The kind that glow in the dark. Surrounded by all those healthy people, I was profoundly aware of my sickness and all that was to come because of it. I knew I was then, and would be, so different from the rest. I felt everything around me was reminding me of how cancer had chosen me, out of everyone else.

As I waited for each girl to check in in front of me, I surveyed the crowd of girls and watched them strap on their bike shoes. I watched as they hurriedly tucked their workout bags in to lockers and then made their way in to the studio.

By the time it was my turn at the front desk, I had removed all my layers, hoping I would fit in a bit better and be more like a pin.

"*HI THERE*! Welcome to the *SPIN* studio! Is it a ride-or-die day or *WHAT*?!" said the receptionist. "What can I get *YOU* for class today?"

If a talking bunny had taken speed, this is what it would have sounded like. This girl was in it to win Employee of the Month. She was decked out head to toe in "SPIN Gear." That's skimpy, shredded, bright colored spandex stamped with inspirational words like Freedom, Love, and Truth on it. Her platinum pony tail was tightly pulled back with a logoed headband and the little star stickers on her cheeks sparkled as she spoke through a fully flexed perma-smile. I could see all her teeth as she chomped on a piece of Strawberry Trident.

"Uh, yes. Yes, it is a . . . ride or die day," I said with limp, lopsided smile. "I'm actually not checking in for class today," I said quietly, trying to be inconspicuous. "I was wondering if I could cancel out my remaining classes for a credit?" I asked in just a whisper, watching as the sparkles on her cheeks came down a full inch.

"Ohhh . . . I'm *SOOOO* sorry! We actually don't *DOOOO* refunds." Her words were arched and curved downwards like a frowny face. "Once classes are bought though, they *ONLY* expire after *NINETY* days so you have *PLENTY* of time to use them!" As her words now curved upwards, they were louder and easily cut through the pulsing noise of the lobby.

"Yeah, I don't think that I'm going to use the classes in ninety days. You see . . ." I didn't want to say it.

"But that's *LOADS* of time to finish your package! *NINETY DAYS!*" She reiterated, like I hadn't heard her the first time. "*WHY* would you want to . . . *cancel?*" She uttered the word *cancel* in a hushed voice like it was a sexually transmitted disease.

"*Mmm* . . . yeah. Um . . . I was just diagnosed with lymphoma, so . . ." I didn't know what else to say.

"Oh wow, oh my God . . . I am *SOOO* sorry," she said with a stutter, as her sparkles now lay flat.

Watching the dramatic change in her demeanor emphasized and underlined how dire my situation really was. Hearing my own words and then watching the reaction that they triggered was like a punch to the gut. Seeing her shock turn to pity made my throat swell and I tried to hold back the tears. I just wanted to get out of there. I wanted to stop feeling so different.

"I'm going to be fine," I interjected. "Totally fine." I ladled on some extra bravado to convince myself as well. My eyes were glassy, and I could feel my mouth quivering. *Don't cry. Don't lose it. Not here. Not in front of all these happy people. I'm going to be fine. I'm fine.*

"Okay . . . let's see what we can do," the receptionist said as studied her computer. "Okay, I could put a *SPECIAL* note on your account to *NEVER* expire," she said. *Never expire. That would be nice. Can I get one of those notes for this body, please?*

"Great. I'll take it," I said immediately, just wanting to get out of the studio.

As I stepped aside to put back on all eight layers, the girl next me unstrapped her shoes.

"Such a great class, right?" she said with a pant.

"Yeah, definitely," I replied, grasping at any chance to fit in with my previous world.

Back outside, I continued to my last and final errand. The Drug Store. As the freezing air blew back my hat flaps and bit my earlobes, I checked the time. *Forty-six minutes left. Battery at twelve percent.* Like a helium balloon loses its height as it deflates, I was now dragging myself down the street to the final item on the list. *Pick up prescriptions.* I had been saving that one for last.

I passed through the doors of the CVS and picked up a basket like a seemingly normal shopper. I was trying to look like I was just in there to casually pick up the regular things like soap, laundry detergent, and birth control, instead of stocking up for cancer and chemo. As I appeared to seemingly peruse the shampoo aisle, I planned my approach. *I'll get the ambiguous items first. Then I can hide the cancer stuff under it. I'll make the pharmacy pick up last.* I was afraid that the people in the store would know that I was sick by seeing the contents of my basket.

In an artful attempt to avoid the other shoppers, I snaked through the aisles like a stealth Inspector Gadget. Under the guise of scrutinizing product labels, I patiently waited for the browsing clientele to clear out of my target areas before I hurriedly heaved bags of Epsom salts into my basket, along with a few liters of Pepto-Bismol, the whole row of travel masks, seven bottles of ibuprofen, and ten handfuls of travel-sized hand sanitizers. As I waited for the coast to clear so I could grab at the anti-nausea bracelets, tongue tablets, and foot magnets, I pretended to scan over the ingredients of the neighboring shelf.

After each hurried hoard, I hid the contents of my basket underneath a value pack of paper towels and toilet paper. I had no idea if this stuff would help me, but it felt good to fill my cart to the brim. Lastly, I dragged by bulging basket up to the pharmacy counter to pick up my prescriptions.

"Picking up for Webster," I said as I poked my head around the tower of toilet paper. After a grueling three-minute wait while the pharmacist collected the last of its contents, he hoisted a large plastic bag over the counter.

I took the oversized bag of prescriptions and immediately wedged them underneath the paper towels. Even though no one was behind me, I tried to shield the view to the rest of the store as the pharmacist scanned each of the items, one by one. He seemed to be moving at an offensively slow rate, like he was truly being paid by the hour. At this rate, he would be a millionaire by the end of the week. *Hurry, damnit.*

With their contents concealed in double bags, I lugged what felt like sacks of sand back to the apartment. *I have twelve minutes left. Battery at eight percent.* It took three trips up and down the elevator to get all my shit upstairs. By the time I staggered into my apartment, I was in a full sweat and panting. I knew I had minutes left before the aches set in, so I frantically tried to unpack and put everything away neatly in its place before I hit the wall or floor, that is.

Finally, I emptied the pharmacy bag out onto the kitchen counter. Out rolled pill bottles, liquid potions and steroid lotions. In every size and every color, they came, rolling out of the bag, off the counter, and onto the floor. It was an entire medicine cabinet in there. It was a fully stocked, geriatric hospital medicine cabinet.

As I bent down to pick up the strewn bottles, the wave of ache washed over my back and seemed to seep from my spinal fluid. My battery had run out, the clock had stopped, and all that was left was the rawness of my reality. *It was just a few weeks ago that I was normal! I was going to work, and the gym, and to dinners out, and I wasn't worried about chemo, or eggs, or long-term side effects, or bodies failing. How did this happen?!*

Anger, Round II

For the second time that day, I lost it. From sheer exhaustion and fear, I was left crumpled on the floor, in heaving, blubbery tears surrounded by impossible-to-pronounce pills with long Greek names. *Is this my life?! Is this really happening?!*

I groped around for my phone to call my parents.

"Oh wow, the bus has really turned around there . . . that didn't take long," I heard my father say as he handed the phone over to my mother. He doesn't handle hysterics very well. My wails were unintelligible, and all my mother could do was know that I was upset, tired, and drained, and try to reassure me, to no avail. There was nothing she could say or do that would stop my bawling screeches.

"Why did this happen to meeeeeeeheehhhheeeeeee? What did I do to deserve thiiiiiiihiiiiiiissss? Why MEEEHHEEEEEEHHEE?!" I sobbed. I pulled out a tissue and blew into it, muffling my mother's coaxes.

"I know, I know," my mother said sympathetically, listening to me cry. "You are going to be fine. Dr. Hodgkin is the best out there. He's going to fix everything. And you know what? I just read an article about *MAT-CHA* tea. You should drink MAT-CHA tea. *They* say it kills cancer."

"Mmm-hmm, okayyyyyyy," I said as I sniffled. My mother was always talking about what 'they' say, whoever 'they' are. But hearing her voice made me feel better, ridiculous suggestions and all.

"Go have a rest. You are tired. That was too much," she said. "Where are you now? Are you home?"

"I'm on the flooraaaahhh," I answered, now full sprawled out on my back.

"Okay. Go have a bath and get in bed. Get cozy. Get some Macho or Matcha, whatever it is. I will see you tomorrow at the hospital, okay? You're going to be fine. It's all going to be fine. Just get some rest."

"Tell her that we got a new housecat, Carolyn. And that we're calling it "Cat." She can meet it when she comes down here," I heard my father say from the kitchen. He knew I loved new pets.

I hung up the phone and stared at the blank ceiling as the aches took over. I could hear Sixth Avenue roll beneath me. Still whimpering, I wiped my wet cheeks with my sleeve as I thought about the next day. It would be my first treatment.

While I lay sprawled on the floor, I was afraid. I just wanted to go back and erase all of it. I wanted to go back to normal. I didn't know what was about to happen in the next six months, but I felt like I was standing in the dark, waiting for the gates of the gladiator ring to open. And I was terrified. I didn't believe I was brave enough, or strong enough, to get through it.

7 What Does Chemo Feel Like?

I met my mother outside the main entrance of the Weill Cornell hospital the next day for my first treatment. With my father back at home, she had driven up from our family home in Philadelphia that morning to be with me. She was standing out front on the phone as she waited for me as my taxi pulled up, and I could tell by the way she hung up that My father was on the other end helping her pass the time. It was a bright, cold day and the winter sun cast dramatic, elongated shadows across the pavement. From the window of the taxi, I could see that she was distracting herself with her phone as she waited, but as my driver came to a jerky stop, her sixth sense made her look up. I smiled with relief as she and her fifteen-foot shadow came toward me.

"Good morning, Choochaa," she said as she hurriedly walked over to greet me. The second my foot touched the pavement, her arms swung around me and my face fit into the familiar nook between her chin and her shoulder. Her scent was a time-traveling tonic that sent me back into my eight-year-old self. My tears came, and I wiped them on her shoulder. I was scared.

"I know, I know. It's going to be okay," she said in the same way she did when I used to stub my toe. "You're going to be fine. One step at a time. Here, let me carry that," she said as she took my bag.

The night before, I had meticulously packed everything I thought I could possibly need into one carryall. Tucked and ordered, my bag held copies of my medical records, insurance cards, a printed email with the time and location details of my appointment, a notebook with scribbles of all my research, and the big bottle of prescription anti-nausea pills that Dr. Hodgkin had prescribed me.

Whereas I had the logistical details tucked under my arm, my mother had two large bags of her own, which were both bulging with all the things someone might need aboard a sixteen-hour flight with a fussy two-year-old. Blankets, games, toys, snacks, an iPad, socks, and even a cooler lunchbox spilled out. Mum was packing some serious heat on the entertainment front.

"Here, put these on," she said as she used her one free hand to slide anti-nausea bracelets onto my wrists. "I swore by these when I got sick on that cruise with your father," she said. She was referring to the time that she got so seasick in the middle of the Atlantic that she had to get an anti-nausea shot in her butt from a member of the cruise's medical staff, which knocked her out for three days while my father wheeled my two-year-old sister around the decks in a stroller. It was an oft-related family legend. "I'm telling you, they work."

"Thanks, Mum," I said as I adjusted them on my wrists, relieved that I brought the full bottle of the prescription pills.

Despite her unwavering good nature, my mother doesn't always think things through, which makes her the best worst person to have around in a catastrophe. In sharp contrast to my father, it's like her logic is the first thing to frantically flee the premises when the alarm bell rings. Like when our cookie dough went down the kitchen drain and clogged the sink, and she unscrewed the pipes to try and clean it out. Rather than lightly flushing the pipes into an empty bucket under the sink, my father had found her in the kitchen stuck in a manic frenzy of catching the overflowing bucket of water and dumping back in to the sink to empty out again. There she was, jolting up and down, back and forth, catching and dumping, in a hysterical craze. The logic had gone down the drain with the dough on that one.

And then, when the back board of our regulation-sized outdoor basketball net shattered into jagged glass all over the driveway, she told us it was no wonder that it broke because it was "supposed to be *inside,"* in the same tone that attaches an eye roll and a ". . . you idiots" onto the end of a sentence.

Despite the somewhat concerning lack of logic under times of stress, Mum was the one that held my hair and rubbed my back when I had stomach flu, brought me beautifully decorated trays of soupy food when I had my wisdom teeth removed, made me drink copious amounts of prune juice while rationing my pain killers after my ACL surgery, and tinkered around with the automatic ice machine for my swollen knee while I yelled from the bed that she was setting it up wrong. And here we were again, about to walk through the doors of another catastrophe. I couldn't imagine having anyone else with me.

"So, how are you feeling, my little honey bunny?" she asked as we revolved through the glass vestibule of the hospital. "I'm okay," I said in a small voice, distracted by the hordes of wheelchairs filled with old people in the lobby, crowding into the patches of sunlight streaming through the windows. "It's the third floor, right?" I asked as I reached into my folder of printouts. I wasn't really asking her for the directions, just thinking out loud.

"Yes. Floor three," my mother confirmed assuredly. "Or was it four . . . ? Are you sure they said three? It might have been four."

"It's the third floor, Mum. Elevators are straight ahead," I said flatly, holding the instructions in my hand.

As we made our way down the large marble hall to the elevator bank, we passed a little chapel room with a sign that read Silence Please. Prayer in Progress. I reached for my mother's arm as she walked ahead, which she naturally and snugly enveloped in hers, and I took a deep breath and closed my eyes. *Give me strength. Please, give me strength.*

Once we were packed in the elevator, my mother and I stood shoulder to shoulder with the other passengers. The crowded air smelled like old skin and dentures. As the elevator rose with a lurch from the first to the second to the third floor, my stomach dropped lower and lower. I could feel the blood pool in my lower abdomen. *Bing.* The cold metal doors of the elevator opened like the gladiator gates I had imagined, and the crowded elevator was flooded with newly sterilized air. I felt like I was on autopilot as I let my mother lead me.

When we stepped out into the hall, we were met with a flurry of nurses and doctors in white coats. Machines were briskly wheeled past us by the hospital staff in scrubs, and everyone seemed to have a clipboard and a mission. Still holding my mother's arm, we jostled through the traffic of the hall to check in at the front desk.

"Porter pickle eye?" the receptionist asked us mechanically, looking from my mother to me.

"A what?" I asked, already confused.

"Do you have a port or a pick line?" the receptionist clarified slowly.

All I could think of was the after-dinner drink of sweet wine served in a voluptuous, curved glass. I was still confused. "I don't know. . . . do I?" I asked as I looked to my mother, who shook her head, signaling "No." Not totally convinced that I didn't have one of these things, I looked back to the receptionist. "Um... How would I know? I was scanned. Where would a pick line be? I'm a patient of Dr. Hodgkin. Maybe he would know?"

I was so on edge and completely distracted by the buzzing activity of the room that I was having trouble thinking clearly. A character trait I share with my mother.

The receptionist exchanged a sympathetic smile with my mother and said that I would know if I had one. "Would you and your sister like to take a seat?

The wait shouldn't be too long." While I ignored the mistake, I could feel my mother's thrill from beside me.

Because of her youthful looks, ageless legs, and our rotating closets, my mother is often confused for a sibling. It happens so often in fact that I'm now used to it. But since it usually puts too much fluff in her feathers, I try to completely ignore it. "Sure, thank you," I said as we turned to find seats in the waiting room.

The last two seats together that were available were in a back corner by an exhausted looking coffee and tea station. I eyed the empty sugar packets that stuck to the dried coffee stains and the strewn little red straws that dangled from the edge of the trash can, like they were wounded soldiers trying to army crawl their way into the garbage bin bunker. "Run for your lives!" they seemed to yell out.

From our seats tucked away in the corner, we had a view of the entire room and while my mother began to set up camp for us with the contents of her bags, I surveyed the landscape.

The droning whir of the main hallway cut through the murmuring conversations of the waiting room. Nurses commuted back and forth across the room, patients were called in and out, the front desk phones rang, and the coffee machine sighed. The lighting was overhead and harsh, and it seemed to exaggerate the thinning hair, shiny scalps, sunken sockets, and deep-set wrinkles of the patients seated around the room.

Most of the patients seemed to be creeping up to ninety. I was by far the youngest in the room. The patients, who often came with a friend, spouse or grown child, sat in silence as they either read the newspaper, knit, or just stared blankly at the nurses crossing the floor or the new patients checking. Everyone in that waiting room seemed so familiar with the busy scene that they even seemed bored, whereas my eyes were wildly trying to absorb it all.

The more desolate souls were parked along the sides of the room in wheelchairs, the same way an overheated car would be pulled off to the shoulder of a highway. These "passengers" were stuck hunched over and muttering to the wall, as if explaining the situation to the cop.

There was an enormous TV at the other end of the waiting room, and an older woman was propped up in front of it watching a muted Tom strap some kind of explosive to Jerry. A woman who seemed to be her daughter sat a few feet away, flipping through a wrinkled, three-year-old issue of *People* magazine.

There were elderly couples who held hands, and entire generations of families waiting. I saw a baby in a stroller get rocked back and forth by one of its mother's hands while the woman dabbed away a dribble from the grandparent's bib with her other. My mother had been taking all of this in as well, and we looked at each other in the way that says, "Can you believe this is happening?"

I felt astonishingly out of place. I felt even more that cancer made a mistake. That I didn't belong there in that room, surrounded by what seemed to be shells of people.

Rows of plastic orange chairs snaked around the waiting room in a way that carved a clear path to two distinct areas: the front entrance where we came in, and a single door leading out. There was a constant stream of nurses crossing the waiting room to make their way from the doctor's offices in the front to the chemotherapy infusion center in the back, and those of us who were in the waiting room were simply sitting on the banks of that tide.

The door to the infusion center was kept closed and locked, but when the nurses swiped their ID cards to pass through it or poked a head out to call the next patient to come on in, I would try to catch a glimpse of what lay beyond. Because there were only brief seconds of visibility into the back room, all I could see was that the lighting was different. It was much softer.

My mother and I waited for an hour before I went up to the front desk to ask for an update. "It won't be much longer," the receptionist said with a smile, when I asked them for an update. "Thanks for your patience, we are a little backed up today."

"Okay, no problem at all. I was just wondering," I said, as I tried my best not to show any sign of agitation. I guessed that the worst thing I could do was to irritate the receptionists because I knew I had a long road of sitting in this waiting room ahead and I needed them on my side.

When I got back to my seat, my mother had unpacked the lunchbox that she had brought for us. Out came protein- and vegetable-packed sandwiches and sparkling lemon waters, equipped with decorative lunch napkins with Christmas ornaments on them leftover from the holidays. She laid the napkin on my lap.

"Here, eat this," she said lovingly.

Right as I was about to take my first bite, a nurse popped her head out of the door to the infusion center and called us in.

"Webster? Webster? Thanks for waiting. Come on back," the nurse said with an Irish accent. She swiftly shook my hand and then my mother's, and as we were taken toward the door, she introduced herself as Judy over her shoulder. Judy wore sneakers and scrubs. She walked quickly and spoke directly. As we crossed just the ten feet to the door to the back, the other patients seemed to know her, and she threw them a quick wave as we passed them.

The door to the infusion center opened with a click, and it was like stepping into an incubator. The room had high ceilings and dim lighting. It was quiet and still. Soft lights reflected off the floors in way that made them glow, and there were rows and rows of cubicles that created small private spaces— incubators—for patient after patient. The only sound I could hear inside what seemed like a "hatchery" was the soft, intermittent beeping of machines as we passed each of the cubicles.

In the same way that I love to look into the lit windows of the buildings across the street from my apartment, I peered into each one of the cubicles to see vignettes of these people's lives. A man sat asleep in a reclining chair with a book on his chest as an IV hung above him. A couple ate their lunch over a table cloth and flowers. An elderly couple tucked under a white hospital blanket were watching an old black and white movie on their private television.

"Here we are, love," Judy said as she escorted us into my cubicle. "Take a seat here, and I will be right back to get us started." She motioned me toward a large reclining chair in the middle. Other than the recliner, the cubicle had two chairs in it, along with a small flat-screen TV, a few piles of neatly folded blankets and pillows, and a tightly packed basket of snacks. A tall IV hook hung above my head, and a curtain was tucked away next to the open entrance.

The first thing I did in the recliner was pull out the leg rest, so my legs could extend out in front of me. I imagined that a first-class cabin on Emirates Airline wouldn't be too far off from this, and I could almost pretend that I was settling in for a flight.

"Okay, here we are," Judy said as she turned the corner into our cubicle with an armful of multicolored bags of liquid. "So, the infusion is going to take about three to four hours, in total. First, we are going to give you anti-nausea pills along with a steroid. And then we start the drip. Your medicine just came up from the pharmacy downstairs, so we are ready to go." She lay the bags of fluid on the counter and moved through the motions with practiced speed, placing this here and connecting that there. I couldn't help but follow along with her nonchalance. As drawers opened and closed, and cords were snipped, I felt like I was sitting at a mixologist's bar watching my cocktail get shaken and stirred.

Once I took the pills, I was absolutely transfixed by the four electrically colored bags on the counter. The blue, red, yellow, and white had the same artificial hues as melted ice pops. Had I been six years old, these colors would have been as tantalizing as ring pops, pop rocks, and sugar dips. And I was curious. *So, this is what it looks like.* The four bags lay next to coiled plastic tubes separated by yellow plastic snaps that looked like little winged bugs. Everything came in the same clear plastic packaging that I used to tear off my toys as a child. As Judy opened each of the plastic encasings of the four bags, the familiar smell of the fresh packaging reminded me of the scented cupcake doll I had gotten for my birthday when I was seven. The one that had her dress flip up to attach to her hat and she transformed from princess to pastry.

I watched with interest as Judy got the needle ready. As I remember it now, I am sure that she purposefully blocked my view of the needle. "Hold out your arm and count to three with me," she said with calm assertion. "One, two, thr . . ." —and with one quick and practiced poke, I felt like a Sharpie marker had been jammed into my forearm.

"We are going to do the blue one first." *Blueberry, blueberry, it's blueberry.*

"Yes. Ready," I said, outwardly confident, yet having absolutely no idea what I was agreeing to. *Holy fehk*, said my inner voice, squirming and squealing.

Judy hung the blue drip bag from the IV above me and plugged the clear plastic tube sticking out of my arm to the long cord on the bag. She tapped the bag twice, set the timer for one hour and told me to press the red call button to my left if I needed anything. Then she left.

There my mother and I were, sitting in our cubicle watching the blue liquid flow from the bag into my arm. Our eyes blinking, afraid to move. With each clicking pump of the automatic feeder on the IV, the blue liquid filled my mouth and nose with toxic, metallic fumes. I could taste it. Every breath I took seemed to evaporate into a burning alcohol on its way into my lungs through my bloodstream, and it felt like I was suffocating. My eyes watered and my toes curled.

"You okay?" asked my mother as the color drained from my face.

"Yup. Good," I replied with a whimper, realizing that there was no way out. Not if I wanted to live.

As she watched my eyes tear and my head roll back and forth trying to shake away the toxic taste, she took my hands in hers. "I just wish it were me," I heard her say quietly.

I could feel the solvent fill every vein in my body. It coursed through my heart and my lungs, my hands, and my toes. Like someone had hooked me up to windshield cleaning fluid, I could almost feel my organs being sterilized and wiped clean.

On the one hand, I wondered how the hell this burning sap was supposed to cure and not kill me, and on the other, I wanted to let it seep into every pore of my body, killing everything in its path.

I closed my eyes to try and give in to the drip. I tried to imagine the medicine traveling furiously through my veins, colliding into the mutant cells and exploding them into millions of pieces. But all I could see was the smoky gray fog of the explosion's aftermath, all I could smell were its poisonous fumes, all I could hear was the sound of static ringing in my ears, and all I could do was watch the blue serum drip, drip, drip into my arm, filling me to the brim.

The first pumps of chemotherapy made me feel like the time I sat at the bottom of a swimming pool. Down and down I had gone as I sunk into its depths, weightless yet sinking. And as I reached the bottom to touch the grainy concrete by the drain, I looked around and was surrounded by the blues and shadows of the water. It was quiet and still under the weight of the water. And I watched the adults hover over me from the sides of the pool, blurred and distorted by the waves on the water's surface. Their silhouettes loomed over the edge to look down at me and all I could hear were their muffled voices, waiting for me to come back up. But under the water, it was so quiet and still. It was eerie and peaceful all at the same time. It felt like I had somehow found a way to slip from reality and float just for a moment on the other side. The undercurrents swayed me back and forth, back and forth, and my palms lay flat like an anchor against the bottom of the pool. I remember that I didn't want to come back up.

This was the first time that I gave in. It was the first time that I truly felt powerless. I had realized the magnitude of the cancer, and chemo, and all the sickness that lay ahead of me, and I knew there was nothing I could do to stop it, or even make it better. Initially, it had felt like defeat. It had felt like cancer had won, and it was going to take me with it, and turn me into just another patient parked against the walls of the waiting room, fighting for my life. I felt that there was nothing I could do but relinquish any grasp I had on my previous "normal" life and let go. This was the first time that I released myself to the currents of cancer.

By the time the first bag was halfway done, I had a woozy, dizzy, heady feeling and the room kept swirling around me. During chemo infusions, cancer patients are encouraged to nibble and sip on anything they can get down. There were minifridges and stocked cabinets filled with apple sauce and pretzels and saltines and ginger ale. For me, the more I ate, the better I felt. And throughout the infusions, it became clockwork to have a lightly toasted bagel when the second red drip was halfway finished, a liter bottle of water had to be emptied no later than the start of the third bag, and I had to pee (fluorescent orange) as the fourth bag started. It was a delicate, critical formula that I learned, and everyone I spoke to that sat in next chair over had their own set of guidelines, like I did.

About forty minutes into that first drip, I finally took my mother up on her outstretched offering of an ice cube-filled ginger ale. The first bubbly sip came as a shock to my mouth. It was like my taste buds were under siege and assumed everything was poison, so it quickly assigned toxic tastes to whatever I ate. Raisins, crackers, mint gum. *Ugh.* Mint gum was the *WORST.*

As we waited for the each of the colored bags to drain into my arm—*How much liquid can one body absorb?* —the floor would periodically seem to drop out from underneath my recliner and I would swirl into empty sickness.

My mother valiantly tried to distract me by telling me stories, trying to force-feed me trail mix and saltines, and manically running around to find Judy every time I thought I was going to puke. The nausea that came with that first drip was the type of sick that one puke can't solve. That shit *lingers.* It even made my eye lids sweat, which burned when it got in my eyes.

I watched my mother as she relentlessly juggled magazines, blankets, and snacks in front of me, desperately trying to make me feel happy, distracted, and comfortable. And as she put on my fuzzy socks and organized a spread of apple sauce and ginger ale, I thought about her. I wondered what it must feel like for her to be here in this cubicle, sitting in her chair and wanting to switch places. And I felt relieved that it was my arm hooked up to the IV, relieved that I wasn't the one on the sidelines, because watching her be sick would have broken me.

Throughout the twelve infusions, friends and family would come sit with me to keep me company. They alternated and would take days of work to be with me for those four hours. Most times it was my mother at my side, or my sister Ashley, who would fly in from London, or Matt, and sometimes it was Bailey or Hallie, one of my closest friends from college. I would send Bailey running around for the bagel and she would entertain the nurses as they gave us both fresh blankets and apple sauce.

One time, a previous, and *incredibly* handsome, former patient of Judy's dropped in on the infusion center to say hello during my drip. He'd had Hodgkin lymphoma too. While I sat there hooked up to my infusion, we had tried to spark a love connection between Hallie and this former patient, to no avail. It seems the chemo infusion center was not the most romantic place for a first date. But how we laughed and giggled, and I forgot, just for a second, about those tubes in my arm.

The underlying point is that it felt good to have people I love be with me during those four hours. They were the best distraction.

When the last bag of that first infusion wheezed its final breath up on the IV hanger, I had felt like I had just chugged a gallon of bleach while doing a few hundred laps in a pool of nail polish remover.

Once I was unplugged and unsnapped from the IV, I leaned on my mother's arm and we made our way back through the harshly bright waiting room, down the elevators, and on to the street.

"Let's walk for a bit," I said foggily. I was feeling drugged and loopy, and just wanted to stretch out my legs and put fresh air in my lungs after spending so much time in the stale hospital air.

"Good idea. Get everything circulating," my mother said in agreement.

From the location of the hospital way uptown on Seventy-Ninth Street, we talked and walked the fifty blocks back down across Manhattan to my apartment. We walked arm in arm, as the alcoholic aftertaste of the chemo sank into the far back of my throat. We called my father and my sister, and I listened while my mother told them how brave I was. I felt drunk and dazed with from the effects of the chemicals in my system. I wanted to keep walking with my mother by my side.

We had walked slowly and peacefully, and it was halfway that we rounded the corner of Central Park that I allowed myself to go back to the bottom of the pool, and sway back and forth with the tides.

When we got back to my apartment, it was early evening. The February sky was already darkening. Matt was home from the office and waiting for us. The energy the steroids had given me was beginning to fade and my eyelids were heavy. My mother tucked me into bed and surrounded me with pillows, as I drifted in and out of sleep.

A few hours later, when it was quiet and dark, I woke up to Matt lying next to me and holding my hand in his firmly against his chest.

8 How to Lose Your Hair in Ten Days

It only took a second refill of chemo for my body to start to reject the smell of the hospital. By the time I got within a hundred yards, it felt like the hospital and I were two negatively charged magnets trying to be forced together. The building invisibly repelled me.

I would coerce my one foot in front of the other, aiming myself toward the front door of the hospital for the next infusion, I listened to my body argue with my head. *Fehk no. No, no, no!* I felt it scream. *I am NOT going in there again. I'm not volunteering to get my insides squeegeed and sterilized again. That shit is poison! Look at what it does! Don't you see?! How sick can I get?!*

"I'M NOT GOING," my body seemed to say as it tried to plant its heels in the ground in front of the hospital.

But my head hadn't gotten the memo. *Get the FEHK in there,* it would say as it dismissed my body's discordance. *Stop whining. It's this or die. Literally, DEATH. Do you want to die?*

"But it's poison!" my body wailed as it was dragged toward the large entryway. "It's mustard gas! Don't make me do it! Please, please, please, don't make me do it!"

Oh c'mon. You are being dramatic. We're going in. Take my hand, stop the whining, and get your ass in there. Stop being a baby and TOUGHEN UP, my mind said as it yanked and pulled my body forward.

My treatment lasted for six months with twelve infusions of chemo, one every other week. I was so fragile the week after chemo that I would have to rest on the bathroom sink after wiping down the mirror after a shower. I would need to hold the arm of the sofa when I got up from sitting to wait for the room to stop spinning. And because my organs were under atomic attack, the blood drained from the outer layers of my body and pooled at my core to protect my vital organs, leaving me an unearthly shade of yellow and gray. One time, I fell asleep midafternoon propped up in bed amid a mound of pillows and woke in the evening to Matt in a suit, just home from his office, with his hand under my nose to check my breathing. My body knew what was happening and it was trying to warn me.

It was after the third infusion that my body started its *physical* revolt against treatment. Like a screaming child throws toys out of its crib in a tantrum, it threw off strands of hair. I was in my morning shower when the hair started to fall. I had felt it slithering and winding down my body. The hair rolled off my back with the water as I crouched over the drain to count the fallen strands. *Two, four six, twelve, twenty, forty. Am I just being paranoid? How much is too much? My hair can't be falling out now . . . can it?! Already?? I'm not ready for this. . . Get back up there. Jesus Christ. I'm not ready for this!*

When I stepped out of the shower, I delicately ran the towel over my sopping wet hair. With one eye only, I peeked hesitantly at the surface of the towel after it left my head, scared to see how many strands were left behind. Out of the corner of my slanted eye, there was a TUFT. A whole fehking TUFT. It had one straggler sticking halfway out of the thatch, floundering in the steamy air as if it was its last valiant attempt to be saved.

"AH!!!!!" I screamed in shock. "AAAaaaAAAHHH . . . aaaaAAAHhhAAAA . . . AAAAAAAH!!!!" In my visceral panic, I bolted from the bathroom as if I could run away from my hair falling out. I frantically dodged and circled the furniture, darting from the living room to the bedroom to the kitchen, moving as fast as someone can move in a 600-square-foot New York City apartment. I seemed to bounce of the walls of my one-bedroom container, not knowing what to do or where to go.

There I was, holding the knotted handful of hair and running dripping, naked laps through my apartment. I was in fight-or-flight mode and my overpowering initial and totally nonsensical reaction was to flee. Flee from my hair falling out. Flee from being bald. Flee from being sick.

After an uncountable amount of blurry and crazed zigzags through the apartment, I stopped to stand still in the living room. I was gasping for breath and trying to fight back tears. "Oh my God, oh my God, oh my God. Holy shit. Holy shit. Holy shit. Fehk. Fehk. Fehk," I said as I stared at the drooping strands in my shaking hand. I was radiating fear.

The room stood still as my brain tried to come up with solutions. *Stick it back in. Wear a hat. Stick it in the hat to hold it in place. Tape. Glue. Wig? How can I get around this?* Realizing I was out of plausible ideas, I stared down at the limp handful of hair and was reminded of the time that I tried to save a baby mouse I had found in the barn where I had grown up. I had delicately laid it in my pocket to ride my bike the half a mile back to the main house, and even though I made sure to peddle slowly so as not to hurt the little mouse, it sadly didn't make the journey back home. I was completely distraught when I pulled his limp body out of my pocket and immediately held a funeral under the maple tree in the backyard for my little mouse, Templeton, complete with flowers and a prayer. Looking at this curled, droopy handful of light brown tufts, it was like I was standing at a funeral all over again.

It was when I was naked and dripping wet in the living room that morning that I realized the inevitable was upon me. It was happening. The effects of chemotherapy were in motion. I was changing. And it wouldn't be long before I transformed completely. It wouldn't be long before everyone could see that I was sick. And I got scared. Because it wouldn't be long before *I* didn't belong. Everything I had built and wanted and dreamed of was disintegrating, the pieces falling through my fingers like my hair in the shower that day. I was starting to lose myself to cancer and there was nothing I could do stop it.

In my attempt to try and fight the unfightable, I went to what I thought was the next best option. *PRESERVATION.*

In a desperate attempt to preserve the hair that remained on my head, over the next few weeks I implemented a few changes. I tried to avoid me, or anyone else, touching my head. I stopped giving big, encircling hugs to my friends when I greeted them for fear that my ponytail would get caught in their embrace and then I'd lose it. I would only go places where it was socially acceptable to wear a hat or a bandana on my head. This ruled out dinners with my friends in nice restaurants, nights out dancing at my favorite downtown clubs, and placing my head on Matt's chest when we watched a movie after dinner.

The list of what I would not do grew as each handful fell.

My efforts to preserve the hair that I had left had a much larger impact that initially intended. As I cancelled plans for dinner and avoided hugs, I pushed myself away from people. It was my first step through the threshold of isolation.

As it turned out, my efforts to preserve were all for naught. They did nothing to slow the increasing numbers of strewn hair I would find on my pillow in the morning, on the bathroom floor, and down the backs of my clothes.

The hairs that clung to the back of my clothes felt like scars. Visible to the world, they told everyone that I was sick. I would frantically brush them off me throughout the day, and was nervous even to stand in line at the grocery store for fear that the person behind me would see all the shedding hair and know something was wrong with me. But most of all, it scared me to see myself disintegrate. It scared me be powerless as I morphed from healthy to sick. And it scared me to give in to what was happening to me. So, I turned to face sickness and cancer head on, literally.

The sheers were warm as they vibrated across my scalp. The long blond hair fell over my shoulders and into my lap. It grazed my hands as it fell in chunks. On the day that I buzzed my head, Bailey and I had picked up a bottle of pink champagne and headed to the salon. I had decided that morning that it was time. I had decided there will be no more handfuls of hair. I had decided to give in, and let the currents take me. And I decided it was going to be a celebration.

I sat in the chair while Bailey set up our phones around us to Facetime with my sister in London and my parents back at home. We explained the situation to Elle, the hair stylist, and she quickly came on board of our impromptu buzz party. She took great care in going slowly, and taking her time, making sure that I was okay. She started on the sides, and moved methodically to each angle of my head while I stared at my changing reflection in the mirror. As she went shorter and shorter with the sheers, I told her to keep going, with Bailey, Ashley, and my parents at my side, at least digitally. It was when the warm sheers crossed the top of my head and the last handful fell that I felt a sharp pull on my chest. It was the same feeling that I get when on a roller coaster and it takes a hurdling plummet towards the ground below.

Looking back, I didn't want to be scared anymore. I didn't want to watch myself change as I twisted down into sickness. But it was when the last of the blond strands fell that I knew I would never be the same. I know realize that the champagne was there to celebrate a crossing, to which I would never be able to return.

After we got home from the salon, Bailey and I sat in the apartment playing with my jewelry as we sorted out my new buzzed look. I hadn't told Matt of the day's activity, and wanted to surprise him, which may not have been the wisest way to handle the situation. I practically scared the living daylights out of him when I sprung open the front door when he got home work. After Bailey had left, we sat on the sofa watching a movie.

He looked over at me and reached for my hand. "You are so brave," he said. "I love you more than I even knew," he said. I was thinking about how cold my head was, and I remember that I wished I could have believed him, because I couldn't see what he saw.

Here is my post-traumatic analysis on losing hair. The trauma was not about the looks, the superficial. I can honestly say that I wasn't super upset about being bald or getting buzzed—which I would eventually do. The upside being that it happened to be hot as hell that spring and summer during chemo and I get frizzy. We know the hair goes because the medicine is working.

But clumps of (staggeringly priced) Frederick Fekkai highlights hitting the shower floor was like watching my body disintegrate before me. Waking up to a pillow of casualties like it was the day after the goddamned Battle of Waterloo was like watching myself decay. And it was scary because it was a reminder that I was sick.

That's why I buzzed it. But then, after the brief moment when I thought I had won the battle and I started to raise that victory flag, vowing with every pull of the rope that I was going to own this shit, it turned again. I was then dealing with a reflection in the mirror that wasn't a reflection of myself, but of someone else entirely. Passing a mirror or a reflective window on the street never stopped being a shock. In that fleeting instant before I realized who it was I saw, I saw this person so different from myself and I wondered what she was like.

Full transparency, I have mistaken myself for a hot lesbian on the street and thought to myself, "Yeah, she's probably checking me out" as I strutted my Lululemon-clad ass to yoga. Inflated ego, *check*.

Egos aside, this intense physical mismatch, among so many other things, made my body so foreign to me. And that feeling of separation between mind and body made me look at myself in a different way, in a new way. It made me curious about who that person was—because damn, it looked like she had a good story.

9 EVERY PARTY
HAS A POOPER

Five days after my third infusion, I was lying in bed
waiting for the sharp line of the morning sun to sweep
slowly across my white duvet and reach my
outstretched legs. April had just ended, and it was a
bright blue day that could have been mistaken for
spring had the smoke and exhaust from the chimneys
and vents on the rooftops across from my building not
been visible to me from where I lay. The windows of
the buildings around me glittered with the passing
traffic below and I could hear the morning rush
beneath me as the world went to work. Tucked away
in my tower on Twenty-First Street, I was sprawled
out flat beneath the sheets waiting for the restless

nausea, relentless, anchoring fatigue, and incurably cold hands and feet to pass. Even though I hadn't moved from my flattened position, my pulse felt strained. I thought that if I lay still and flat, the blood would have an easier time finding its way around my body.

Twenty-three more hours. I had one more day with the side effects. *One more day. Tomorrow it will be gone. Tomorrow I get my body back.* Like waking up after a flu breaks, the Day Sixes throughout chemo reminded me how strong the body can be. How resilient it is. *We made it. We made it through another one.* But now, I had to wait for the vortex to pass.

Ambling up onto my elbows, I tried to raise myself out of the fog and the walls around me seemed to swirl and bubble. It was like reliving the ugliest hangover for five days in a row, except this time there was no champagne, no tequila, and no dancing to substantiate it. My bones hurt. My hips ached. My body felt stiff and strained.

I slowly propped myself up on my pillows determined to get myself through my now normal morning routine. Since I had stopped setting an alarm for work, I had implemented my own structure in my own little realm above Twenty-First Street.

I usually woke up around 9 AM. Instead of prying open my heavy eyelids to race to the shower and out the door to the office, I would now sprawl myself out to take up the entire surface of the bed. After I enjoyed about thirty minutes of a good sprawl, I would get out of bed, pull the shades all the way up, and shuffle my way to the coffee maker. There, I would make a latte with foamed milk. Sometimes, I'd even sprinkle cinnamon on the top.

I would take my time foaming and stirring. While the coffee machine would drip, I would stretch. I would have a leg up on the counter and one arm reaching up to the top of the fridge. Once the latte was ready, I would take it back to bed.

I would prop myself up with pillows and tuck a heating pad behind my neck. I would stay there for about an hour, reading, talking on the phone, or scrolling through news updates and emails. It was during this time that I would usually check in with my body. I would ask it what it wanted to do that day. Sometimes, it would be a walk through the West Village. Sometimes, it would be a seat in the sun. Sometimes, it would be straight to the sofa.

The key here being that I was at the mercy of my body during cancer. I was at its beck and call. So, I gave in to it. I let it tell me what to do and when to do it. I had nothing to lose except this body, so I gave it total and complete control. I was learning its language, with each drip of chemo.

On this morning, as I waited for Day Five to end, I wrapped my cold hands around the warmth of my latte. I picked up my phone to see if I could rejoin the world, at least as an onlooker. I scrolled through it with one eye shut thinking I could trick my brain into thinking I was sleeping and not scrolling. Since scrolling screens and chemo nausea don't mix, I typically went days without checking my phone, which made me feel even more removed. *Bing, bing, bing.* My emails loaded one after the other and the notifications came sliding down my phone. One caught my eye. It was a calendar reminder for an engagement party for friends of me and Matt. "Calendar Alert. May 7, 2016. 4 PM. You are confirmed 'Attending.' Event in five days."

As both eyes burned into the screen, my brain suddenly realized that it was staring at a screen and cold, wet nausea consumed my abdomen making the insides of my checks swell and water. It felt like my intestines had dropped even further into my groin.

Now I felt so sick that saliva was filling my mouth and I forced myself to swallow, which made me gag. I thought of the party. *How can I go like this? What will everyone say? Will I be that sick person? The one with no hair? What will they think of me? How could I possibly have a good time like this? I am literally disintegrating. And drooling. I'll ruin the appetizers.* I had RSVPed months ago when I thought I'd be fine, and that if not, I would deal with it later. Well, it was later.

I ran my hand over the top of my buzzed head. The hair was short and strong, and soft like velvet, but when I looked at my hand it was speckled with tiny hairs. I turned slightly to see my pillow behind me and it was a sprawling surface of casualties. I had gotten used to seeing little pieces of myself trail behind me.

Can I even go? Dr. Hodgkin said I should avoid germs because my immune system is compromised from chemo. That's it. I can't go. Doctor's orders. But . . . then does that mean I must be apartment bound until therapy is over? Am I going to be a bubble boy? That's five months of seclusion! Five months of isolation! That can't be normal. Or healthy.

I'm going to go. And I won't touch anyone. I have nothing to hide. Everyone can just deal. This is the situation right now, and this is the best I can do. I'll put on makeup. No, what am I thinking? I can't go. I don't have eyelashes.

The debate went on for days. By the time Thursday rolled around, Matt had listened to the brunt of it and held his ground on a "Do what you are comfortable with" position and "Either way, you decide." I didn't know what to do.

On Thursday night, my best friend Bailey came over to help me try on outfits for my potential debut on Saturday. The deciding rule was that if I had nothing to wear, I wasn't going. Matt had come home from work early by chance, so he automatically got roped in to the fashion show. There I was, trying on my entire closet and marching all my favorite dresses out into the living room for the judges.

Now, you would probably have expected these two to tell me everything looked great, that I had nothing to worry about, that I looked totally normal and was an even *better* version of myself, right? No. That's not how this went, and I have a pinky swear promise to prove it.

When Bailey and I were in boarding school together, we sometimes would entertain ourselves by getting on the scale to weigh ourselves in the medical center. At boarding school, we had to get creative with our recreational activities, and the scale was like going to Home Depot for a self-renovation. The medical center was conveniently located just a short one hundred feet from the entrance to the dining hall, so it was an easy stop. We stood up on that thing one afternoon after field hockey practice and the scale read my weight at about seventeen pounds over my usual weigh-in. Seventeen pounds on a five-foot-seven-inch frame was catastrophic. It was amazing that I was walking and not waddling.

Horrified, I looked at Bailey. As she held her hand over her mouth, she told me "It is all muscle" and not to worry about it. I tried to convince myself that she was right or the scale wrong, but I was having trouble thinking clearly with the waist band of my jeans digging so deeply into the rolls of my stomach. *Maybe I won't have that third bagel today*, I had thought as we headed in to the dining hall.

Later that following summer, after I had been constrained to a diet of fish and vegetables at home, Bailey and I were looking back at pictures while we visited each other during our summer vacation. Like the inflated blueberry that was Violet Beauregarde in *Charlie and The Chocolate Factory*, I must have taken up half the pictures. My swollen cheeks squeezed my eyes into these tiny beads and I could almost hear the strained grunts of my pants through the plastic film as the seams clung desperately together. We were in hysterics looking at these pictures while we sat on her bedroom floor that August, funny only because I had since slimmed back down.

"It's muscle?!" I screeched as Bailey's appeasing, well-intentioned but false claim floated to the surface of the pictures. Through her laughing gasps and as she wiped her tears off her face, she promised always to tell me the truth from there on out.

Now Bailey and Matt sat like judges on the living room sofa as I paraded around all my favorite party outfits.

"Nope. No. Definitely not. That does not look the same," Bailey said as I stood in my favorite cocktail dress. "There's just something about florals and a buzz cut. Just doesn't work. Next."

Matt tilted his head, trying to see her point. "I like that dress, though."

"Let's try monochromatic," Bailey suggested. "All one color. Let's see what happens then."

While she helped me sift through my clothes, I passed over all my go-to favorites and it was like I had outgrown or out-changed them. Like that time when I sat playing with my dolls as a child and it suddenly became unfun. In one sharp minute, the game had ended though I still wanted to play. Something had changed. Their made-up voices sounded strangely forced, and no matter how hard I tried, I couldn't bring the pretend back. It had gone, and I didn't know where or why.

Bailey and I landed on a navy blue fitted dress, a crewneck with long sleeves. I call it my SCUBA dress because all I needed were a pair of flippers and some goggles to be able to scour the ocean floor in it.

"That's IT. That is a TEN. Love it, love it, LOVE it," Bailey said emphatically. "That is the LOOK. You look like a badass. The buzz, the blue, it's PERFECT."

Her enthusiasm was contagious. "You're right . . . I AM a badass," I said.

I marched my badass self out to show Matt and he nodded his head again, not quite sure what he was looking at. "I think I like them all, but this shows off your butt." Badass, indeed.

"Okay then. I'll go. It will be fun! I'll get a little break from the apartment and feel like myself for a few hours, right? A few hours with all my friends. It will be good for me," I said as clasped my hands together and did one last twirl in front of the mirror to check out my backside. It was decided. I was going.

Late that Saturday afternoon, Matt, Bailey, and I piled in to the car and headed to the party. It was out in the suburbs of New York City, where the houses had manicured hedges, front gates, and stone features. The towering oak trees out front swayed their draping branches as if they were fanning the rolling lawns, screened porches, and big black Range Rovers parked in the driveways. The sun was starting to set as we drove up the driveway of the house.

I remember the feel of the front door of the house on my palm. I remember pausing to listen to the happy, laughing voices on the other side. Bailey and Matt had gone in with the gifts and I had taken my time getting out of the car to arrange my coat and prepare myself. I had said I wanted a moment.

I remember slowly stepping over the cracks in the brick walkway that led up to the framed front door of house. The air was cold on my buzzed head and my fitted blue dress seemed to stifle my swiftly beating heart under my coat. *I have nothing to hide. This is*

the best I can do. This is me right now. Be brave.
They are going to look. They are going to ask. They
will get used to it. The shock will pass. Like it did for
me. Just be brave.

I anticipated the weight of the stares, the
attention, the sympathy, the sadness. But most of all,
I anticipated the feeling of being naked, exposed, and
broken in front of a room full of one hundred healthy
people. I felt like a patched together version of myself
with my red soled heels, my fur coat, and a small
clutch stuffed with the pills that I had to take in a
few hours. I felt awkward and deformed.

The last time these people saw me was when I had
long, blond hair, a big laugh, and boundless energy.
What will they think of me? What do I think of me? I
don't feel even feel like me. I could barely recognize
myself. I looked at the glossy sleeve of my fur coat
and felt jealous that it had hair and I didn't.

My flaws were visible. Branded with my cancer for
everyone to see, I waited outside the door, listening to
the laughter on the other side. *Be brave. This*
condition is not my fault. I have nothing to be
ashamed of. This is me, right now. I have nothing to
hide.

I took a deep breath. *One, two, three, and push.*

Walking into the room full of guests, I used every
ounce of my courage to keep one foot moving in front
of the other, and not crumple under the nearest tufted

seat cushion. I crossed the living room to greet the hosts and could feel the stares around me. *Be calm. Be brave.*

"CC, we are so happy you are here," Mrs. Host said, as she gently held my shoulders. "What a shock it was when we heard. I am so sorry that you are going through all of this."

Mr. Host then appeared next to his wife and was nodding his head as they both looked upon me with sympathy, in the same way someone would look if I had said my dog died.

"How are you *feeling*?" Mrs. Host asked.

It was this question that became the hardest for me to answer in social situations. This question prompted a choice. I could either answer with the uncomfortable truth and say that I've been leaking toxins out of every hole in my body for weeks or I could tell everyone what they wanted, or *needed*, to hear.

"I feel really *good*. I feel strong," I lied. I just wanted to help Mr. and Mrs. Host manage their sympathy and get myself to the bar.

In perfect stride, Matt swung in from the left just then and whisked me away to the drinks tent. "How are we doing?" he asked.

"Such a strange experience," I said as I filled my glass of white wine with ice. "I'm not sure how to handle it exactly." The truth is that I was still adjusting to the weight of the stares and trying to digest the scene. I wasn't sure how to act or behave in this new, foreign body of mine.

"They are all so happy to see you, Ceece. They love you. Just tell me when you've had enough though and we will go, okay? Seriously," Matt said reassuringly. It felt good to have an out.

"Okay. I can do it. It will be fine. They'll get used to it. Walking in was the hardest part. It will be a nice break."

The next hour of cocktail conversations circled around three things: my health, other people's cancer-related stories, and heaping, steamy mounds of unsolicited advice. I was led over to be introduced to the one other cancer survivor at the party. Then Wacky Uncle Number Three rubbed my head like I was Buddha, and then Mr. Horn-rimmed Glasses tapped my wine glass and asked, "Should you be drinking that?"

Uh YES. YES, Sir, I definitely should be drinking this in order to get through this conversation. Should you be smoking that cigar? I'm sure it's not good for that high blood pressure of yours. Looks like your face is going to explode.

As I circled through the crowd, I started to grapple with the situation and I started to understand. As Pink Blazer with the Hermes Scarf was telling me all about her father's prostate cancer,

I understood. As Mr. Madras Shorts and Knee Socks got out his phone to connect me with his friend who performs vitamin infusions, I understood. As I Can See Your Nipples You Should Have Worn a Bra asked question after question on how I got diagnosed, how "they found it" and what were the first signs, I understood. I watched guest after guest close like a clam as I passed, and I understood.

They saw themselves in me. They saw their worst fears come alive, in me. Sickness makes people feel uncomfortable. My cancer reminded the people surrounding me at the party not that it can happen to anyone, but that it can happen to *them*. It reminded them of their own fragility and their own pain. And I listened. I understood that no one knew what to say or how to say it.

While I was sick, there were friends who didn't call, who wouldn't call. But I understood. It was scary, and it was sad, and they felt like there was no right thing to say.

While I circled the terrace of the party, I saw that my cancer triggered a variety of reactions. It was over talked. It was unspoken. It was happy and relieved. It was terrified. Surrounded by all those friends and acquaintances, I felt out of place, alone, and unsure of myself. It was like I was just getting used to the controls of a new deformed body and I had to pretend that everything was not just normal, but that I felt *good.* And *strong.* Because that's what they all needed to hear. I could see it.

At the party that night, I watched as my friends' eyes would try to discreetly scan my buzzed head and the bulging purple scars on my neck and I could see that my appearance scared them. In the same way that someone pretends not to notice the green piece of spinach lodged in your canine, I repeated the diagnosis story again and again while they briefly skimmed my scars with careful curiosity. So naturally, after I finished my first watered down white wine, I started talking about my scars *for them.* I even encouraged them to touch the baby duck fluff on my head. All of this in a blind attempt to alleviate the discomfort that surrounded me.

As I tried to make everyone around me as comfortable as I could, I began to understand that my cancer was going to be a solitary experience. I realized that it was impossible for anyone else to understand what this was like, how it felt. The saddest part for me was the feeling that I had to cut away the ropes from those closest to me. Matt, my mother, Bailey, and that room full of people. That I had to sever the tethers despite how badly they wanted to come with me. Like a lonely boat floats away from the crowded dock, or a balloon from its tightly bound bunch, I felt like I was watching them wave from the distance as I disappeared over the horizon and floated calmly and irreversibly out into the oblivion.

"You ready to go?" Matt said as he slid his arm around my waist. He knew I was exhausted.

I nodded, and we made our way back through to the entrance.

As he slid on his coat and helped me into mine by the front door, he said, "I love you, Ceece. I'm with you." But I had never felt so alone, as I felt my boat drifting away from everyone and everything I loved.

10 Ex Corpus

I accepted that cancer was going to be a solitary experience. Despite my friends and family wanting to be there for me, I came to realize that it was impossible for them to come along. Even by doing all the right things, like sending flowers and notes, it was impossible for them to feel what this felt like. They couldn't know the gravitational lurch in my stomach when those first handfuls of hair lay limp in my palm, and they couldn't know what it felt like to plead with a God as the scanning machine orbited around me, or know the burning acidic difference between the red chemo drip and the blue one. They couldn't know what it felt like for me to watch my whole world shift and sink around me while I clung onto the fraying rope of normalcy in an attempt to keep from going under.

As the infusions went on, and the more I retreated into isolation, I struggled with my relationship with the world, specifically acknowledging and accepting the support around me. How I related to my world had changed in one fell swoop with the cancer diagnosis, and I was unsure how to interact with it anymore. In one camp, I didn't want to pick up the phone and talk about how I was feeling. In the other, I didn't want to be alone. This dichotomy was mirrored in those around me. Some friends didn't call, couldn't call. They didn't know what to say, or how to say it. I knew it was scary for them too, and I knew they were unable to be there for me.

Other friends would encourage me to go to support groups and they would connect me with their other "cancer friends" so we could "share experiences" and "talk." This sounded terrible to me. I couldn't imagine anything worse than hashing out chemotherapy with a stranger. So further and further, I repelled into my own little universe.

I tried not to think about how different my life was before the diagnosis. I tried not to feel displaced and forgotten as I scrolled through rows of smiling, laughing faces tossing around their full heads of hair on Instagram. I tried to remind myself that my treatment would be over soon and that I would be able to get back to normal again. I would get my body back again. This became less and less believable the farther I sank into treatment.

Cancer patients struggle with the feeling of isolation. For me, in dealing with cancer at a young age, it was feeling that life was going on without me that was the worst part. While no one knows exactly what to say or what to do when someone they love is in the middle of cancer hell, I found comfort and support in little pieces of normal. I saw the gifts in the seemingly mundane.

The best phone calls were when Hallie was walking home from work and wanted to tell me about her day. The best emails came randomly and described a morning, a thought, a memory. Sometimes these had nothing to do with anything, but were just people giving me a little piece of themselves. The best texts never demanded a response, but just told me that someone was thinking of me, or that they had laughed when they were reminded of one of our adventures together. It was the simple, little pieces of normal that made me feel less lost, less alone, more loved, and more included.

On top of this growing sense of isolation, my own self-acceptance was sinking fast as I continued through treatment, as if into a bubbling, consuming pit of quicksand. This made me want to hide even more, because I didn't see myself as myself. This wasn't me, but a someone else. A temporary, someone else.

I rejected the new form that I was taking. Not only did I feel isolated and separate from the world, but I was a bald, tired, aching, seemingly crippled version of myself. Going outside of my apartment to get a manicure was considered a big day. Just putting pants on was a workout that required a gasping rest on the corner of the bed. My days had me moving from my bedroom to the living room and back again. Ordinarily I went no further.

I watched as my veins started to turn bluer and bluer through my increasingly translucent skin. And with each passing infusion, I got more and more exhausted. I don't mean "go take a nap" exhausted, I mean that I could feel my body getting tired. Tired of it all. Tired of feeling. Tired of being scared. Tired of being too weak to move. Tired of struggling for life. It was telling me to stop. I could hear it.

I was retreating deeper into a strange alternate universe that I carved out for myself, separate and isolated from the world that buzzed beneath my apartment window. One night, about halfway through treatment, I found myself alone in the apartment and restless. Matt was working late, and I had the apartment to myself. I was in Matt's oversized college sweatshirt and sweatpants, shuffling around the apartment in my socks, while carrying around a half a glass of red wine, the one I had been milking for hours. I found myself pacing from room to room, moving from bedroom to living room and back again. This is where 600-square-foot apartment gets problematic. Had I been in a large house, the pacing would have been classified as wandering, but since I was lapping my route every ten seconds, it made me feel even more uneasy. I felt lost and desolate.

With each step, I blamed cancer for taking my life away from me. I felt sorry for myself that I wasn't out with my friends but alone in the apartment, in an oversized sweatsuit and socks. I felt angry that I didn't recognize my reflection in the dark windows. I felt angry that cancer kept me here in this cage, angry that it had put everything on hold, worried that it all wouldn't be there when I got back. Cancer and chemo had stolen my hair, my energy, my job, my dreams, my purpose, and my sense of self, and had given me this in return. I felt robbed and victimized. It only took a couple more laps for the anger, the sadness, the fear, and the resentment to blend into numbness. I was tired of feeling.

I gravitated to my bedroom, like a mechanical android, as New York City pulsed beneath me. I opened my closet and stared at the clothes hanging. I started taking everything out, slowly and calmly. I wasn't sure what I was trying to do, but I did it methodically, like I was opening the drawers up for the first time. One by one, I pulled out every tee shirt, every dress, every sweater, and every pair of pants. One by one, I tried them on and stared in the mirror. I just couldn't stand to see a sick person anymore. Looking back at myself, I squinted, searching for something else to see, other than a cancer patient.

I slowly went from shirt to shirt, changing out pants, slipping into my tallest heels. Each time I faced the mirror, I looked at my bald head, my thinning face, the dullness in my cheeks. To me, I was unrecognizable. An unearthly version of myself. As I folded back the cuff on my sleeve, I looked at the bright blue veins in my arm.

My whole life I have had the ability to create my own reality. I realized this power when I was eight, while I was playing tag with my friends during recess in third grade. I had gotten bored with the game and was trying to find other ways to stay engaged and involved. Not wanting to just quit the game and stop playing, I thought of a better version, for just myself to play. I switched from being a little girl in a tunic uniform and penny loafers to being a velociraptor. Different from the original, boring game where we were just regular humans, I imagined I was running around with a bunch of dinosaurs instead. This was much more fun.

I made sure not to make my dinosaur-like movements too obvious, to still blend in with my friends and not give myself and my secret game away. However, when the game ended, and we were called back to our desks, my friend Amy leaned over to me and said, "This is really weird, but has anyone ever told you that run like a velociraptor? Like in Jurassic Park? It's really cool. I wish I could run like that."

I quietly shrugged it off and thanked her for her compliment, but inside I was reeling with excitement. I had discovered my very own superpower. The imagination.

As I stood in front of the mirror, dressed in all black, my figure stretched up from the floor of the mirror frame to the very top of it. The light was behind me and left shadows on my face. And I began to see something else. Instead of being sick, I was bold. Instead of being weak, I was brave. It was as if I was slowly placing panel after panel, plate after plate, around me, protecting myself from sickness, and cancer, and chemo. With each plate, I took myself out of my body and turned myself into the mechanical android that I needed to be.

The blue in my wrists and the matte of my skin showed me something else to see. But most of all, the panels and plates protected from feeling. No more drips, no more loneliness, no more fear, no more anger. I wanted just to let there be nothing. I wanted to go numb and give in to what was happening to me. I wanted to give in to the tide. No more fighting. Let it take me. Take me out of this body. Make me into something else. Ex corpus.

By the time Matt came home, I had already fallen asleep. I felt him crawl into bed next to me and reach for my arm as he usually did. And I remember that I moved away from him, so that he couldn't reach me.

11 It All Started with Deodorant

Throughout the first few infusions of chemo, I never cried. I never felt scared. And I never believed that I could die. A vivid memory throughout the experience, however, was how everyone else cried for me, felt scared for me, and thought that I was flirting with Death himself, standing on the dimly lit threshold of his creaky front door. I could see it on their faces when I told them of the diagnosis. I could feel it when they hugged and held me for longer than usual. Their fear and sadness seemed to radiate through the room even as I reassured them that "I was going to be fine."

I felt like I was constantly reassuring everyone around me. On the rare occasion when I did socialize, most people would usually compliment my daring new haircut if they hadn't yet heard that I was sick.

"Oh, thanks. I actually have lymphoma," I would say, feeling the need to clarify. They would gasp. "But I'm going to be FINE," I would add immediately, hoping swiftly to replace the air that had escaped their obviously seized lungs. Many people seemed unable to follow me over to the second part of my sentence. The "I'm going to be fine" part. Everyone would always circle back to the cancer part with questions. *Interesting* questions.

For example: "Oh my God, how did that happen?" was always an interesting one to try and answer. In the privacy of my head, I ran through many responses dripping with sarcasm, which I kept to myself. *You know, I remember the very moment when my cells went on strike. One said to the other, let's fehk shit up. Yes, I know EXACTLY how it happened, when it happened and why. I'll be sure to tell the scientists and researchers all over the world that we have finally found the answer to the mystery of cancer.*

"Oh my God, how did you know you were sick?" was also always a fun one. Depending on my mood, I would swing back and forth from: *"Well, what I thought was a little cold turned in to CANCER. YEAH. Better check yo'self"* to *"I felt like I was going to DIE at four o'clock EVERY DAY."* What I said aloud would depend on the reaction I decided to invoke. Both renditions of my story—the minimalist and the melodramatic—were equally true.

The most telling inquiry was this one. "Are you going to be all right?" It was telling because it was proof that they weren't listening to me—because I had just said that I was going to be fine. This was proof that they couldn't hear the other end of the sentence. It was proof that they believed cancer led to inevitable, tortuous, disintegrating death and they feared the worst for me.

The questions and the reactions that had surrounded me at the beginning of my cancer treatment started to haunt me. *Why wasn't I feeling as scared as everyone else? What was I missing? Is there something someone isn't telling me? Everyone around me is so upset for me, fearful for me, sad for me. Why do I not fear inevitable death? Why haven't I cried?*

The only thing that was eating at me—disintegrating me, literally—was the treatment. Despite my assuredness that "everything would be fine," the side effects of chemotherapy were wreaking havoc on my body. And I could feel every bit of the destruction. While everyone was focused on the cancer, I was battling the treatment.

I was on the phone with my mother one morning when the chemotherapy took its final toll. "How are you doing, lovey?" she asked. "You know, I was thinking about that rash on your neck that you just got, and I read something saying coconut oil could fix it. Or was it tea tree oil? I have to check. Whatever it was, there is some kind of natural oil that might help. I will send it to you."

Chemo had recently branded me with a raging reactive rash that encircled my neck like a scaled red snake. Dr. Hodgkin has said it was my immune system reacting to the therapy, and to go see a dermatologist. The dermatologist had given me a topical cream, but it hadn't worked. Since I couldn't take a pill, all I could do was try and deal with the intensely burning, itching, fiery scales on my neck and shoulder. It was excruciating. But it wasn't the rash that was the final straw. It was my words. Chemo started to take away my words.

"Mum, I can't take it anymore. I can't sleep. It's not even just the rash. Everything hurts. It's like my bones are . . .*pulsing.*" I floundered trying to recall the word *throbbing.* It felt like it had appeared in my head and then vanished as it slid across my tongue.

"No, not *pulsing.* . . . What is the word?" I tried again. "My bones . . . My bones are . . . Fehk. WHAT is that WORD?! Mum! I can't remember the word! What is the fehking word!"

"You have *aches?*" she said, trying to fill in. But by that point, I was in a full-fledged panic. I realized that I was losing my word recall. Chemotherapy was taking my words away from me. Cognitive effects were a real side effect that I had known about since I had initially researched chemo after being diagnosed. The list now popped up in my head (miraculously, since I couldn't recall anything else it seemed), like it was being pulled from a filing cabinet.

Cognitive impairment. This was what was happening. I really was losing brain power. I was losing my mind—actually. Instead of bursting into tears at this recognition, I remember that I started trembling. My voice shook as I clutched the phone to my ear, desperate for consolation.

My mother said, "Calm down. Deep breaths. You are going to be fine. It's all going to come back when this is over. You know what? Your sister sent a name of a homeopathic doctor in New York. Or was it a naturopath? I can't remember, but maybe you should give her a call? She might be able to help. Why not, right? At least it might make you feel better."

"Okay," I said as I ran my hand over my head. I had nothing to lose. No more hair, just my words. My mother gave me the number of the homeopathic doctor and I called that day to set up an appointment. I spent the rest of the day trying to recall the words in an attempt to keep them all active and inside my head. As I opened the fridge for lunch, I would say, "Fridge," as if I was teaching a five-year-old the names of the kitchen appliances. "Sink." "Spoon." "Magnet." I thought by saying all the words I could think of, they wouldn't go away.

That night, I told Matt about the day's vocabulary catastrophe. "I think going to see the naturopath is a great idea," he said. "What have we got to lose, right? The last thing we need to be doing is worrying out about side effects, right? Maybe she can help." I loved how he said *we* instead of *you,* including himself in my plan.

I moved my dinner plate from off my lap, as I sat nestled in the corner of the sofa. "Will you take out the trash and do the dishes?" I begged, reluctant to get out from beneath my furry throw.

"Looks like you haven't lost all of your words," he mumbled as he got up from his spot next to me.

A few days later, I was sitting across from the naturopath in her office. The room was tranquil compared with the hospital that I was so used to by now. It had a sofa and a desk instead of the cold, sterile exam chairs and beeping machines with long cords. I felt like I was in a friend's living room.

"Let's go over your food diary," Dr. Naturopath said as she sat in a chair across from me with her iPad on her lap. *Food diary. No doctor had ever asked me what I was eating. I had succumbed to the organic movement, but I had never considered that certain foods had certain uses and effects.* She was professional but warm. Serious but soft. I had provided her with the lengthy intake questionnaire that outlined four days of my eating habits along with all my recent blood work and medical records. We reviewed my symptoms and side effects in conjunction with my behaviors and personality traits. We discussed the physical effects of cancer treatment *and* the emotional ones. We sat for two hours as she explained the ways in which I could help support myself through chemotherapy, and then together we designed a plan. Her suggested solutions were natural and practical, and they didn't involve prescriptions or pills. They *supported* the chemotherapy, and didn't fight it.

Dr. Naturopath's approach was one that took in to account all aspects of health and the body, and she had simple solutions for my seemingly impossible problems. As chemotherapy progressed, the list of side effects only grew and my treatment options had gotten fewer and fewer. Like Epsom salt baths for bone aches, coconut oil for skin rashes, yogurt for yeast issues, and healthy oils and fats for my word recall. Yes, my body needed chemotherapy right then to rid itself from the cancer, but there were things I could do to help the medicine work and to protect what I could in my brain and body from the atomic bomb of therapy. This wide lens approach to my health opened a door in my treatment. And it all started with deodorant.

The first thing Dr. Naturopath had told me was to stop using my high-powered, aluminum-packed deodorant and switch to a natural brand. Cancer loves aluminum, and I was literally slathering it onto the lymph nodes under my arms.

Back in my apartment, I stood in front of my medicine cabinet in my bathroom. *If deodorant is bad for me, what else in here is bad?* The bathroom raid turned into a full-blown apartment raid. I read every label on every bottle and filled a garbage bag with paraben packed shampoos, phthalate- and sulfate-rich creams, paraffin-laden soaps, and toxic cleaning products. With one eye shut, I turned to my face creams and makeup last. It physically hurt me to throw away my two-hundred-dollar face cream, but if it had formaldehyde in it, it had to go. I basically performed an exorcism in my apartment that day, and rid it from everything toxic.

Once I detoxed the apartment, I thought perhaps I should cleanse the emotional as well. Throughout my diagnosis, I had become aware of the idea of a "Type C," which is a cancer prone personality. For those searching as to "why cancer happened," there is a theory that there are a set of shared personality traits that make you more susceptible. Personality traits such as a tendency to repress emotions, and to take on more and more responsibilities even when they cause you long-term stress, adversely reacting to life changes, worrying often and excessively about others, and feeling the need for approval from others. *(Psychology Today)*

To me, there were emotional *causes of* my cancer as well as *because of* my cancer. I wanted to help myself clear away the emotional garbage, and support myself emotionally through treatment. I knew I needed help in this, and was learning that I couldn't do it alone. So, I found myself a psychologist, one that specialized in cancer and trauma.

Psychological Counseling

One of the earliest ways I chose to help myself get through cancer and chemo was to begin seeing a psychotherapist for counseling once a week. I realized that I had six months to focus on myself and felt that this would be a good time to try and sort out whatever the hell was going on in my head. I didn't go to my psychologist with a list of problems in hand that I was hoping to solve, just with an urge to explore how certain things happened, what they meant to me, and how to cope. I became fascinated with exploring why I am the way I am through my weekly sessions. After a year of therapy, I find it difficult to understand why everyone doesn't go.

As the chemo infusions continued, I kept seeing my psychologist. However, other issues were appearing that seemed to demand a different kind of help, in addition to counseling. I was struggling with sleep and with an empty void of energy. I was tired in so many ways. I felt so sick all the time. My sleeping cycles were distorted, and I felt stagnant and slow. So, I started to research ways to reboot my energy, and found craniosacral therapy.

Craniosacral Therapy

Craniosacral therapy focuses on making sure your body is moving fluids efficiently, especially in the channels around the spinal cord and in the skull. The pulse of fluids can be disrupted due to various traumas, like injury, repeat motion, sickness, and so on. Practitioners believe that craniosacral manipulations can improve the circulation of the cerebrospinal fluid, improving overall circulating and energy flow throughout the body.

I went in to my appointment not knowing what to expect, which was good because my placebo effect is very powerful. Like I'm the one who could get drunk on nonalcoholic beer—*that* powerful.

The practitioner placed her hands over all the major joints and hinges of my body while I lay on the table. She placed extra focus on the top of my neck and the base of my spine. While her hands moved ever so slightly around the base of my skull, she asked me whether I sleep by a window or if I feel anxiety in the mornings or evenings. When I said, "Yes," she adjusted the placement of her hands. I left the office not feeling any different than if I had laid on the floor for forty-five minutes, a little dizzy and a little sleepy. But I went to bed that night and I can't tell you the last time I'd had such a great night of sleep. I attributed this to the craniosacral therapy.

While in the later stages of chemo, a good night's sleep is incredibly rare. I woke up feeling refreshed and excited for the first time in months. I felt calm and relaxed at the same time. It was the best I had felt in months. It was magic. Ever since then, I go every few weeks for craniosacral work and I get the same reaction every time. It's basically witchcraft, and I highly recommend it.

It was during one session of craniosacral therapy, that the practitioner identified that I had a buildup of tension throughout my body. She said that she could feel that I was tensed and braced, which was limiting the circulating of blood and oxygen through my body. She recommended acupuncture and massage to help relieve this physical and emotional tension. So, I gave it a try next.

Acupuncture

HELL YES, acupuncture. A practice that has been around for thousands of years, why wouldn't I give this a try? I am now totally addicted. What does it do? Anything you want. Literally. How did it help? I could feel knots and muscles twitching with each poke and prod of the hair-thin needles.

If you are afraid of needles, don't worry, you can't feel anything but relaxation.

The acupuncturist identified pressure points to relieve specific stresses and pains. Once the needles were in position, I was left in the room for twenty to thirty minutes or so, a sufficient period for the needles to do their thing. Sometimes treatment felt like a warm wave washed over me, as each muscle and nerve seemed to relax. I would often drift into a light sleep during my acupuncture sessions, which, for someone who was not sleeping, speaks to how powerful the effect is. Highly recommended.

For me, the combination of counseling, craniosacral, and acupuncture led me to a new level of self-awareness. I was becoming more and more aware of my physical and emotional self. I was learning that the two are powerfully connected, which is something that I had never considered. My career in pharmaceutical advertising had taught me the power of the pill and how a groundbreaking medicine can solve all your problems. But once I was faced with that medicine, I learned that emotional effects come with it.

I was living proof. We are not just physical bodies, we are emotional beings, and our feelings, stresses, drives, and worries affect us more than I had known.

I set out to explore this new connection I had made between mind and body through different modalities. I had learned about the Feldenkrais Method from the craniosacral practitioner I had seen. She had recommended it as a natural way to help relieve the body aches brought on by chemo.

The Feldenkrais Method

The Feldenkrais Method is a subtle therapy that promotes both physical and emotional self-awareness. By performing small movements, the method aims to "reteach" the body to become more aware of itself and the ways it can move most efficiently. Because "we move according to our self-image" (Moshe Feldenkrais), the emotional self is often affected as a result, making it more aware of bad habits and tensions, helping it become a better problem solver, and enabling a deeper understanding of the self.

During my session, I lay on a flat, cushioned table while the therapist made small changes to my body's position. I was supposed to feel the effects of these adjustments resonate throughout my body. I didn't feel anything.

Through her coke bottle glasses, Ms. Feldenkrais would look up from her place underneath my left leg and ask, "How's that? Do you feel it? Your hip just adjusted itself back into alignment."

Hmmm. Nope. I must have missed that, I thought. "Oh, yeah . . . I think I felt it," I said aloud out of pity. I couldn't wait to get off the table.

Maybe I was expecting to hear pops and cracks, or something at least a little more dramatic, or perhaps my physical self-awareness was underdeveloped, and I was trying to run before I could walk in the proverbial sense, or perhaps it was because I had to pee very badly the whole time I was on the table, but I found the experience underwhelming.

Feldenkrais wasn't for me at that stage in my therapy, but I would consider giving it another try.

During Feldenkrais, I found that I had craved the pops and cracks that I imagined to be chiropractic. I went to a chiropractor next.

Chiropractic Adjustments

I found myself on the chiropractor's table after I had a knot the size of China under my left shoulder blade. It was a knot that would periodically wake up with, and it would stay for weeks. I was told that it was a build-up of tension and a side effect of the steroids that I was being given. It limited my neck movement, which limited my joint movements, making me feel uncomfortably stiff, sending me to go get adjusted, hoping to relieve the tension in my upper back and neck.

Those first pops in the chiropractor's office were life changing. I felt like my entire spine got put back into place. I got off the table feeling a whole foot taller.

Honestly, I could lay on the chiropractic table every day, but I hold off and go once every few months. For me, it was a revolutionary means of relieving my stiffness during treatment.

Moving from Feldenkrais to chiropractic adjustments addressed my acute physical ailments, but I knew I had to find a headspace that would help me with the emotional effects of therapy. In pursuit of helping myself through it all, I turned to meditation, because, well, that's what everyone around me was telling me to do.

"Have you tried meditating?" they would ask, when I would tell them how much the hospital repelled me, or how I couldn't sleep, or the looming dread that would encircle my abdomen before each infusion, or how the acidic drip felt as it traveled through the plastic port in my chest to my bloodstream. "You should try it."

Based on how intense the physical and emotional effects of chemotherapy were, I was a little bit cynical about the idea of "focusing on your breath" to remedy them all. But I gave it a try, just in case it was more significantly powerful than I believed.

Meditation

Throughout chemo, everyone I ran into—friends and practitioners alike—kept harping on the magic of meditation. In the beginning, I really struggled with sitting still for the ten to twenty minutes of the sessions and often found myself peeking at the clock to see how much time was left. Perhaps it was my choice of audio tracks that put me off it. I listened to guided meditations designed expressly for people undergoing chemotherapy, and each time the voice on the audio asked me to imagine the "magical fluid" as it "glided through my veins" I almost puked.

I responded better to the idea of taking ten minutes to check in with myself to scan my body from head to toe and ask myself "How are feeling today? Any concerns today?" I loved the idea of counting breaths and rhythms.

I am a person that quite likes being inside her own head, so I created my own space to do just that. Some days are harder than others when it comes to meditation. With anxiety specifically, an image that helped calm my mind was imagining myself at the bottom of an ocean. As the waves ripple and bounce on the surface, I was calm and quiet, swaying with the tides as my hands rested on the sandy ocean floor. The practice of dedicating ten minutes each day to grounding my body and mind in this manner really did help me address many of my challenges throughout treatment, cynical or not.

Through meditation, I learned how to be aware of my physical body and my thoughts. I learned to speak to my body and listen to what it had to say. Through meditation, I learned, even more, how connected the mind is to the body. The practice has solved many of my emotional hurdles throughout chemo and beyond.

Meditation naturally led to yoga. Yoga was like a moving meditation, and it felt good to stretch and move my aching, tired body.

Yoga

I found that doing yoga a few times a week cleared up many of my physical symptoms, and even a few emotional ones. Once I found myself spontaneously crying on the floor while splayed out on the floor lying in Savasana (corpse pose) at the end of my practice. As I left, wiping the tears from my face, I felt like the giant weight had lifted off me. Also, I found that yoga clears the mind. I was able to focus on myself in the yoga studio. I was able to move and stretch, slowly and calmly. I found that this helped my body feel *used* through the stagnancy of sickness. It got blood flowing to my fingers and put color back in my cheeks.

Very soon, I found myself looking forward to going to my weekly classes. Throughout chemotherapy, as well as after, there was something incredibly healing about being in a quiet room with quiet people just trying to be better.

At the beginning of treatment, I would get plugged in to the chemo drip every other week believing my body had failed me. By the end of the experience, I started to see that perhaps *I* had failed *it* instead. I used to push my body. I didn't listen to it. I forgot about it. And I thought it would always be there, at my disposal. I learned that I had to give back. I had to listen. Because this body would not be taken for granted. And if I could help myself through one of the most toxic and rigorous treatment protocols currently being used, why wouldn't I?

Through my travels in the salt rock crystal-lit offices of complementary and alternative medicine, I gained recognition of just how intricate, complex, and powerful we really are. Because the human body is one hell of a force.

12 THE MATT CHAPTER

Relationships are hard. Throw cancer into the mix, and they get even harder. By the time I was halfway through therapy, the emotional stress of sickness and the physical effects of cancer and chemotherapy seemed to have taken their nonrefundable toll on our relationship.

Every morning, Matt used to kiss me goodbye before he went to work.

"I don't want to wake you up," he said when I asked why the kisses stopped.

I used to get a big, gripping, happy hug when he stepped through the door at night, briefcase swinging on his shoulder.

"I don't want to hurt you," he said when I asked where my hugs were.

He used to ask me to come meet him and his friends when he went out for drinks after work.

"I know you are tired," he said when I asked where he had gone.

We used to go on dates every weekend, just us. We used to go dancing. We used to see our friends. We used to stay out late. We used to sleep in. We used to walk around for hours a day, exploring the city. We used to hold hands when we fell asleep. We used to try out new restaurants, sit at bars. We used to plan last-minute trips to go skiing and loved to be the last on the mountain at night. We used to get dressed up and go to parties. We used to reach for each other in the middle of the night.

It didn't all stop in one day. In the way that a leaky bucket of water empties drip by subtle drip, our intimacy went unnoticed until it was gone. The last drip fell on a Saturday morning in April. It was bright and cold outside, which made me feel warm and cozy shuffling around the apartment in my socks. I had woken up to make coffee and left the door to the bedroom open, hoping to wake Matt up in the same way Folgers coffee wakes up an entire family, dogs included. But instead of those blissful Folgers smiles, I was met with "Damnit, CC, shut the door! I'm sleeping!" It was 9:45 AM.

Matt had gotten home in the small hours of the morning the night before. As he had tried to discreetly slide into bed, I had been woken up by the rustle of sheets and the movement of the mattress as he turned on his side, facing away from me. Even though I knew he was exhausted from his grueling work week, I had hoped to have a nice morning together, just like we used to. We would slide around in our pajamas, make breakfast, and as the bacon sizzled, we wouldn't be able to keep our hands off each other.

On this morning, at his angry command to shut the door, I went into the bedroom and immediately opened the blinds. I pulled them all the way to the top of the window frame. Matt was sprawled out in his boxers when the light smacked his face, to my satisfaction.

"Oh my god. Stop! Let me sleep!" he whined as he pulled a pillow over his head to block the light. With a grunt, he turned to face away from me again, as I stood over his side of the bed thinking of how to get him up. So, then I jumped on him, which used to work so well that it got *everything* up.

"Ugh. Get off," he mumbled, annoyed. And with one small push and a grumpy groan, he rolled over and I tumbled from my perch on his hips onto my empty side of the bed. I stared at him from my place across the sheets as he fell back into a snore. Each of his breaths seemed to bring me closer to the realization of where I was, where *we* were, right then, at this moment in our relationship.

While I sat in a bath of Epsom salts smothered in rash cream, he was going after his next promotion. While I tried to wear lipstick instead of mascara when my eyelashes fell out, he got all new suits. While I was throwing back naturopathic supplements and green juices, Matt was throwing back beers with his friends. While I was having seven different types of vegetables in my morning smoothie, he was crushing a pint of Ben and Jerry's ice cream after dinner.

Here I was doing everything I could to help my body get healthy, and it seemed as though he was doing just the opposite. Here I was living a shadow of a life, and it felt like he was doing everything ten times more. Here I was left behind, and he was moving forward and faster. And now, here I was, getting pushed away because I couldn't keep up.

As I lay in my place across the sheets from Matt, my fears that cancer would eventually make me lose love seemed to take on a physical shape and barge into my reality. From the beginning, I had felt guilty that Matt had to be with me on this one. I felt sad that the person he had fallen in love with had changed forms on him, into a version unrecognizable. And I felt responsible for deterring the path of our happy, hopeful relationship. But most of all, I had worried from the very beginning whether he would stay. And if he didn't, or couldn't, I had promised myself that I would understand.

Looking back, I now realize that in the months prior, I had been pushing Matt slowly away, back to his regular twenty-nine-year-old life. Every time he reached for me, I had pulled back. Every time he told me how brave or strong I was, I didn't believe him because I couldn't see what he saw.

In the beginning, cancer and chemo and sickness weighed on us as one. I could tell that my worries were his. I could see that empathetically he felt what I felt. It was like he was taking on cancer too. And I couldn't watch it. I soon felt guilty that Matt saw my sickness as his to bear, and I knew that he needed to be released from its grasp. He needed a reminder that he was the healthy one, that this was my battle to fight. I saw that he needed a reminder that he was young, with lots of life ahead of him. Cancer hadn't chosen him.

In the same way that I resented cancer for taking away the life that I had planned, I was terrified that Matt would resent me for taking his. I was terrified that by letting him come with me through cancer, it would kill everything we had built together, just like the chemo. So, I had given Matt back his life separate from mine, slowly and systematically. I had tried to push him out of my boat by encouraging him to continue on with his plan, and by telling him that it was totally fine for him to work late or go enjoy himself. That he actually *needed* to get out and enjoy himself.

I encouraged Matt to go play squash and golf. I told him that it was okay if he worked late. I told him to go be with his friends. I told him that I didn't mind if he wasn't home with me all the time. I told him to not worry about me. I encouraged him to go take care of himself too, in a way that I couldn't.

These one nights seemed to lead to three and four. And now, I felt like he was always working late, or had a squash game, while I was left alone at home. He had work dinners, sports games, and weekend activities. And I had fallen behind.

On the Saturday morning in April, as I lay in my place across the sheets, I realized not only the presence of this great divide between Matt and I, but that I had built it, brick by heaving brick.

Folgers coffee, you might have a new commercial.

Sometimes, from our window overlooking Sixth Avenue, I would watch Matt walk down the sidewalk next to our building with his briefcase at his side. He would cross the street and merge with the flow of people as they walked to work. And I was jealous. I was jealous that he got to rejoin the world, and I was left home alone, with my weak, sick, tired body. I tried to imagine what he might be thinking whenever he saw a pretty girl on the subway. Did he look at her? Did he feel guilt and sadness because of my sickness? And as I indulged these daydreams, it seemed that the dead weight of fear and responsibility was breaking us.

By the time I got halfway through chemotherapy, Matt and I were leading two different lives. We had morphed into two different people, living in two different dimensions. As any cancer survivor can tell you, the isolation is one of the stresses of sickness. I realize that I helped feed that loneliness during my sickness by pushing those closest to me away. Unfortunately, Matt got the brunt of it. I was trying to push him out of my boat and at the same time wondering where the hell he was going. And he was trying to keep our lives as normal as possible, letting me be on my own when I asked to be, afraid of treating me like the sick person that I was.

Relationships naturally have arcs and dips. A relationship with cancer involved fused the arc and dip as one, and sent Matt and I to either side of the spectrum. It was a tale of two cities. We were inversely related. The deeper I sunk into sickness, the more Matt rose to assume the role of my caregiver. The more Matt was my caregiver, the less intimate we were. The more I changed into a version unrecognizable, the more I isolated myself. The more I pushed him away and told him that I was fine, the lonelier I got.

It wasn't until I was a year into remission that I learned that the intimacy hadn't really gone. It had changed and morphed into a version unrecognizable. It didn't disintegrate away, but grew in different, unexpected places instead. Intimacy can be many things. And for me, for us during chemo, it was when Matt simply refused to get out of my boat. It was in all the things that he did for me, that I never knew about. I still don't know what was written in all those emails he wrote to our friends, describing each milestone in my therapy and telling them how proud he was of me. I still don't know what he saw when he told me how beautiful I was as I sat in the infusion chair covered in hospital blankets.

It was when he sprinted the thirty blocks uptown from his office when he couldn't get a taxi and I had my first appointment. It was how he sat with me for every trip to the hospital and back. It was how he would let me yell at him for not throwing the milk out. And it was how he would check my breathing when I fell asleep sometimes.

Looking back, I can see that the intimacy had never left us. It had just morphed into a version unrecognizable, for the time that it had to.

One year after my last infusion, Matt asked to marry me in a small, dimly lit restaurant in the West Village of New York City. He was so nervous that his hands were shaking and all he could do was put the little velvet box in front of me and search my shocked face for any sort of a yes-related reaction. After all the life that we had gone through together, he asked if he could spend the rest of his with me. He told me he would do it all again. When he told me how brave I was, how beautiful I had become, and how he would do it all again if we had to, I believed him.

When we met with the priest at a tiny church in SoHo before our wedding ceremony, we told him our story. The priest took a small pause, as his eyes rested on the marriage vows. "In sickness and in health, you two," he said as he nodded his head with silent approval. "And you have been tested already."

13 SO, THAT HAPPENED

For me, the aftermath of cancer was the hardest part of treatment. Throughout the six months of therapy, I had figured out how to settle in to sickness. I had armored and braced myself for that next drip, that next day. Like a machine, I had kept my head down and my feet had moved methodically one in front of the other. To survive, I had chosen not to feel and not to think about what was happening to me, but to just give in and let the current take me.

When the day came that I was told I was in remission, it was like I had crashed up on to a sandy, gritty beach, gasping for air. I had thought that I had finally been set free. The doctors handed back my body and I thought that I could move forward with my life and all the plans that I had put on hold all those months ago. I could go back to work. I could stop being an android and reenter civilization. But there was a catch that I had not anticipated. The body I got back had been irreversibly changed, and no one had introduced us.

It was as if the doctors were sending me on my way in a stick shift, and I only knew how to drive an automatic.

On the day I was told I was in remission, I sat waiting for the results in an exam room with my mother. I'd had my final scan a few days before. As I sat on crinkly paper on the exam table wrapped in a purple hospital gown, I wrung my clammy hands together and hoped to God that He had heard the prayer I'd said in the scanning machine: "Please make it all be gone. Please don't light up like a Christmas tree. Please let this be over."

I seemed always to speak to God when I was lying inside that beeping scanning machine.

We sat in silence, my mother and I, looking at each other apprehensively, as questions about the scan results ricocheted through my mind. *What if the chemo didn't work? What if they found something else? What if it spread? What if it's not over? But then, what if it* is *over? What do I do then? Where do I belong? How do I go back to normal? So much has happened. So much has changed. . . . How has it all changed me?* Every outcome seemed equally daunting.

"Congratulations, CC, your recent scan showed up negative," Dr. Hodgkin said as he stepped through the exam room door. He was carrying my results in his hand. "You are officially in remission," he said proudly and conclusively as he displayed them.

As I processed his words, my eyes welled with tears. Then I could do nothing else but jump off the table and hug Dr. Hodgkin right then and there in my gown. It was over! I had made it. I had tumbled out the other side of cancer and now all I had to do was to pick up where I left off.

I was overcome with relief. *No more poison, no more sickness. I got my life back. I just got my life back. I can go back to normal. Everything can go back to normal.* In the same kind of happy blur that happens when the ball drops at midnight on New Year's Eve, I pushed aside all the worry about what would come next and just let myself bounce up and down with joy while the proverbial confetti fell around me.

When we got back to the apartment, Matt was home early from work and together, we called my father, my sister, and everyone close to us to tell them the news. That night, my mother, Matt, and I celebrated with a dinner at home.

"Oh good. Thank God. I thought you were going to look like an egg," My father said over the phone when we told him I was officially in remission and there would be no more chemo.

My mother made my favorite roast chicken, and we sat together at the table recounting memories over the past six months. The circling through doctors, the phone call during my meeting with the agency partners, the biopsy surgery, and the hurling of the juice boxes, the first treatment, and the forty-block walk back home afterward, the first buzz cut, the cocktail party, and all of the strange reactions I had gotten there, the rashes, and the word loss, and all the support I had found to get myself through to the other side. The memories were all tinged with the same bewildered hue of "How the hell did that happen?"

I slept soundly and peacefully that night, awakened only by Matt's hand reaching for mine. The next day, I called Human Resources at the agency to tell them the news of my remission and that I was cleared to come back in eight weeks. When I hung up the phone, I felt like I was reconnecting all the cables of my previous, precancer life.

Everything was going back to normal. In the following days, I fell back into my idea of what I thought I should be doing and saying. I fell into the motions of taking care of my healing body, getting ready to go back to work and rejoining the world. But strangely, rather than basking in the glow of my remission, my thoughts were starting to slowly swirl and swell. The worst of it came at night.

At around 3 AM, the worries would slowly trickle in and pool at my feet. I would look at the different aspects of my life, scout out everything that was out of my control, and become overwhelmed with panic. Everything out of my control would taunt me like a deranged child taunts a caged animal. *How am I going to manage the demands of my job? What if I can't do it? What if I can't keep up? What if I get sick again? How did I even get sick? How did cancer even happen? Why did it happen to me?*

Does Matt still love me as much as he used to? Or am I irreversibly changed, forever broken? Will he ever see me the same again?

When will my hair come back? Now that cancer is over, what am supposed to do now? Where do I belong now? What happens next, now that it's over? I fought so hard to be here, now what? Does going back to my old self make it all worth it? What if it doesn't?

I had an overwhelming fear that reentering the world as my previous, precancer self wouldn't justify my walk through hell and back. It wouldn't make it worth it.

As the questions swirled and pooled in my mind night after night, there was nothing else I felt I could do but close my eyes, try to sleep, and try to keep moving forward hoping that the anxiety would pass as I regained my strength over the next few weeks. Unfortunately, this ostrich-in-the-sand approach only fueled the fire and eventually pushed me to the brink of a total existential meltdown. If there was a time to have a mid-life crisis, this would have been it.

The more I tried to act like everything was normal and fine and good, the worse I felt. On a morning after an anxiety-ridden, soul searching, tossing and turning night, I woke up to the revelation of a hazy blue late-summer sky through the open windows of my apartment. I groggily looked at my phone for the time and realized that I had been asleep for only a few hours.

Ding, ding, ding. My phone went off as more text and email notifications continued to pour in. The previous week, Matt had sent out an email to all our friends letting them know the news of my remission. I scrolled through the growing list of responses that had been piling up in my inbox over the last seven days. "Congratulations!" the emails read. "So excited for you!" "When can't we see you!" "We can't wait to celebrate with you! When are you free?" One after the next, day after day, the notes had come in. And with each one, I seemed to slide inch by inch back under my duvet, unable to respond to anyone. *When am I free? Isn't that the question of the fehking hour?*

I was just so *tired*. All I wanted to do was to disappear. I knew I needed to figure out how to face the world again, but I felt like I wasn't ready. I felt like I was this strange hybrid breed, caught between sick and healthy. Outwardly, I had been cleared of cancer and set free to resume my life. Good as new, right? Internally, I felt like I had been through the tumble dry cycle of hell.

Trying desperately to make myself feel better, I was determined set out to do all the things that I normally liked to do before, and then during cancer. I got up. I had a good sprawl in bed. Then I registered back in at Spin Cycle and took a class in which I ended up just peddling the bike to my own beat. I got acupuncture. I organized myself for work. I wanted to belong again. I went through the motions of rejoining my life, but I felt numb to any emotion other than anxiety.

Wasn't I supposed to feel excited and happy and hopeful after beating cancer? Any YouTube video or morning talk show will tell you that. Wasn't I supposed to celebrate that the cancer treatment was done for good? Wasn't I supposed to rejoice that I got my life and body back? *Joy. That's what I am missing*, I decided.

There was only one way to infuse a good shot of joy into my newly resurrected life and that was to do two things: Throw a party, and get some hair. So, I did just that. Perhaps hosting a Wig Party would snap me back into my previous reality, transforming me from this numb blob I'd become to my recognizable self. *Semi*-recognizable, due to my florescent pink bob.

Two weeks later and in full regalia, Matt, Bailey, and I piled into a cab to go downtown to the commemorative wig party celebrating the end of my cancer. It was the hottest day of the summer, but I didn't care. I had a hot pink hair on my head and it was the first time that people on the street weren't looking at me that pitiful "You are sick" way; they were just looking at me in that "Why are you on the streets in a florescent wig at 5 PM on a Thursday" kind of way.

Everybody I knew came. The party was filled with people who gave me so many hugs and so much love. I was enjoying myself so much that even I forgot, for a moment, about all that had happened. I was just happy to be out with my friends, holding a beer, and telling stories from when we were in high school. That night, Matt and I came home and sat at the kitchen counter while I made tea before we went to bed, pink wig and all. We recounted stories from the night and made ourselves laugh. The party had been an incredible release for the both of us.

As we headed off to bed, I went into the bathroom to take off my wig and wash my face. I studied my face in the mirror. As my buzzed head became visible again in my reflection, the spindly teeth of anxiety resumed their grip on my stomach. As the wig fell to the floor, I was dropped right back in to my reality. Here I was facing the aftermath of cancer. Here I was trying to pick up the pieces after cancer had exploded it all into gazillions of sharp pieces, pretending that I was the same and that everything was normal and that I was fine. Even after I kept trying to do what I used to do, go where I used to go, and be who I who I had been, I realized the sheer impossibility of it all. Everything that had happened just couldn't all go away now that is was over. It wouldn't all just go away.

I realized that I had been in costume not only at the party, but in the weeks after chemo had ended. Like a cast of characters after a play, I was stripping off a performance. I was playing pretend that none of it had happened. And scarily, that game of make-believe had made me feel more like myself than I had in months. But it wasn't the truth. The truth was that cancer was not going to let me forget. The truth was that there was no going back.

Yes, the hair would come back. Yes, my eyebrows and eyelashes would grow in again. Yes, my body would biologically normalize and regain its physical strength after twelve infusions and six grueling months of chemotherapy. But the truth was that I was irreversibly changed. I wasn't the same person that I was before cancer, and I had yet to meet this newly formed, raw replacement.

This insight was a terrifying moment for someone like me who had always relied on maps and plans to navigate her world. I felt like I was in uncharted waters, in a foreign ship, with no idea how to work the steering wheel, and no idea where to steer to. Cue total and collateral existential crisis.

Rejoining my previous life by forging ahead like a machine and doing all the things that I used to do only highlighted, with a (fluorescent pink) highlighter, that I had changed. It threatened that I might not belong in my old life anymore. The ground had just fallen out from beneath me and I was terrified about what was to come next.

That night, Matt asked why my hands were so cold. I couldn't even formulate the words. Where could I even begin? I was in a total body paralysis, so I told him the AC was on too high.

Rejoining life after cancer was like a test, one that I failed at miserably. It was like the universe was testing me on what I had learned throughout the experience and it was seeing how I applied those learnings to my new cancer-free life. In my case, on my test, I tried to chemically engineer the ways cancer had changed me. I tried to pick and choose the impact it had on me, and make them work to my advantage.

SO, THAT HAPPENED

Spoiler alert: This approach does not work.

Eight weeks after my remission, still in paralyzed shock, I went back to work at the agency. I was determined to resurrect my previous life and all the plans that I had had for myself. I was determined to keep moving forward, keep marching onward, hoping everything would sort itself out and my previous self would eventually reappear from out of the fog.

Initially, I tried to rejuvenate my previous ambitions in the office. I wanted to succeed again. I wanted to belong again. In my first weeks back, I dove right back into the long days and the late nights of the endless demand of the advertising world. I wanted to show everyone that I was better than before. I wanted to prove how cancer had changed me and I wanted to preassign the ways it had made me smarter, tougher, and wiser. I was still trying to control the uncontrollable.

In the office, I got a myriad of reactions to my cancer. There were a few new faces scattered among the familiar ones. Most people avoided the subject of where I had been for the last six months entirely and pretended that they didn't notice my buzz cut and the scars on my neck and chest from the surgeries. Others praised how much energy I had and commented on how it was like nothing had ever happened to me, how it was like I had never left. Meant as a compliment, I would thank them and each time the words would fall from my tongue, something in me would stir and become unsettled.

As the weeks turned into months, I dove even deeper into work, desperate to prove myself again. Despite my previous promises that I had made to myself to take care of myself and my body in order to handle the demands of the job, I began to slowly fall back into old habits of skipping meals and working late. Eventually, I stopped making it to my yoga class because I just couldn't get there in time. One after the next, I stopped prioritizing appointments with all the doctors and resources that had helped me get through treatment. It was my way of conforming to the pressures of my life back at work, conforming to the plan that I had designed for myself, cancer or not. But unlike years past however, I would wake in the middle of the night with drenching night sweats and a rapidly beating heart.

As I look back, I can see that I was trying to forget all that cancer had taught me. It had no place in the world that I was in. There was no tolerance for it. So, I pushed it all away because I wanted to keep up again, to belong again. I knew that there was no room for weakness, and there were no special exceptions. So, I made myself forget.

With each passing day in the office, working on the same projects with the same teams of people, I began to feel more and more at odds with where I was and what I was doing, which only made the anxiety worse. I wasn't feeling more like myself as time went on; I was feeling less and less like myself. Everything I would have been excited about previously now seemed mundane and pointless to me. Everything that I had wanted for myself now seemed a waste of time. I struggled to find the same joy I used to have swinging from the limbs of the corporate tree. It was like I had fallen out of love with all the dreams I'd had. Everything that had made me recognizably myself before cancer was different. Cancer seemed to have stolen from me my ability to dream and be excited about the future.

As the anxiety grew and I felt more and more out of place after cancer, I started to recognize that I wouldn't be able to march on like this too much longer. The life that I was desperate to resurrect was starting to creak and sway. It was going to break.

The nails, bolts, and beams didn't come crashing down in one swift realization. It happened gradually, through one comment, one email, one meeting, one look. And I just couldn't force it any more. I couldn't find the passion again in what I did. I couldn't get excited for the future anymore. I couldn't force the script on how cancer changed me. And most of all, I couldn't justify being back in the same place, doing the same thing as before. It just wasn't worth it. I had fought too hard.

And I had known this from the beginning—from the day I had returned to the office. Like a broken relationship that goes on for too long, working at the advertising agency was no longer right for me. Once I admitted this to myself, I cleared off my desk, packed my things, and left, leaving all the plans I had made, all the dreams I'd had for myself since childhood, at the bottom of the recycling bin with the previous week's project status reports.

I took the down elevator, crossed the marble lobby, and walked out the front door.

It was late morning on a Tuesday in March that I sat on a bench by the Hudson River, warming my face in the steam of a cup of undrinkably hot tea from the coffee shop across the street. I watched the waves of the river as they rolled and glided across the water's surface. They reminded me of the time that I sat at the bottom of the swimming pool and swayed back and forth, back and forth with the tide. I had given in and let them carry me as I sat on the grainy concrete by the drain, surrounded by the shadows and the blues of the water. It was so quiet and still under the weight of the water.

I took a sip of the scalding hot liquid and felt it burn my tongue and then warm my throat as it swirled its way down. I felt the cold air on my fingers and the warmth of the cardboard cup in my hands. I felt my heart beating and its pulse, pulse, pulse through my body, down my legs. I felt my weight on the bench and the hard, frozen ground beneath the soles of my shoes. And it was the first time that I was proud of this body of mine. I felt the life pulse through me. And I felt calm. I felt young. I felt strong. I felt my own energy and I knew I would only get stronger if I nurtured this body of mine.

We've fought too hard, this body of mine and I, so we are going to make it count. We are going to make it worth it.

CODA

Me again. As I was writing the last chapter, it occurred to me how perfect it was that the book was ending there. With Chapter 13. You see, the number thirteen and the date are meaningful to my family. But then I wanted to explain why. Hence, I've written this coda.

Here's the story.

My grandfather was one of the thousands of Allied troops that stormed the beaches of Normandy during the Battle of Dieppe in World War II. This was one of the bloodiest battles in the war, and a military fiasco. Many historians believe the troops were sent to their deaths by the generals due to the overwhelming numerical and geographical advantage held by the

Germans. While thousands of soldiers lost their lives as they crossed the beach that day, my grandfather managed to come out of the battle unscathed, only losing a toenail.

A single toenail was shot clean off.

By the time the conflict was over, my grandfather had been captured and become a prisoner of war. He was freed on Friday the thirteenth of November.

In many ways, cancer made me feel like I was in a crowd of thousands hurtling across a hellish beach, ducking fatal bullets, and fighting for my life. I came out the other side with just a two-inch purple scar on my chest, and my life intact, when so many others don't. Cancer comes in so many forms and breeds, with so many outcomes. I feel like the bullets missed me.

Throughout my chemotherapy infusions, I sat in the infusion center's waiting room a total of thirteen times. And each time, I was reminded how lucky I was. Because it could have been so much worse. It could have been catastrophic. But for some unknown reason, I came out the other side with just one scar.

This begs the question, why didn't the "bullets" hit me? Why was it me who got to the other side? More importantly, how can I honor all those who didn't make it?

I didn't come out of cancer knowing the meaning of life. I don't have all the answers. I didn't meet God.

And things still scare me. Cancer didn't tell me who I was, what I should do, and how I should do it. Having cancer was a process. One that taught me not the meaning of life, but the magic in it.

I have scars. And it was *rough*. Emphasis on the rough. But I choose to look back on the year I had cancer with fondness, and a little bit of Friday the Thirteenth luck. There was magic in the smallest moments. Like when my best friend sat next to me in the infusion chair and made me laugh, and when Matt climbed in my boat to come with me, and I fell in love with him all over again. There was magic in exploring a new way to care for myself, in discovering all the hidden angels that helped me get through to the other side. There was magic when my dreams for myself got shot to hell in a cannon, and I got a better version instead.

Because there was magic in what came out of all these things, I believe that honoring the way cancer changed me is honoring the experience.

As I write this coda, it is November thirteenth and I am thirty years old. I was lucky to have been diagnosed with a treatable cancer and have my life at my feet. Maybe, hopefully, there will be decades more to my life, and I will simply look back on the year that cancer happened as a chapter in my story.

As I said, I don't have all the answers. But here are a few of the guidelines that I have applied to my life during my year in remission, after cancer happened, which I believe merit sharing.

Simple Life Guidelines

- Respect the body. This comes first. Always do what feels right, what feels healthy. Cancer taught me that there will be no more pushing past my boundaries to meet the needs of someone other than myself. There will be no more putting myself aside. When my body says enough, it's enough. I am honest, open, fearless, and unapologetic in this.

- Be open. During my cancer treatment, I explored anything and everything that could help me get through it. I was desperate to support myself in any way I could. In this, I had to step beyond all the pills that I wasn't allowed to take, and I discovered myriads of ways to help my body. Some of it worked, some of it didn't. I learned to be open to trying the unconventional. Open to new experiences. The effects were undeniable.

- Take risks. Cancer lit a fire under my ass to take risks and act now. Not because I didn't know how much time I might have, but because I *had* time. And I had to make it worth it.

\- Never hate a Monday. Cancer taught me to never want to hate a Monday again. It just wasn't worth it anymore. I wanted to stop counting down the days in a week, waiting for the next promotion, or the next raise, the next weekend, the next year. I was always thinking about what's next, never what's now. Cancer woke me up to the idea of *now* by turning my predesigned plan on its head. It made me reorient my passion and my purpose, made me ask, *What makes me happy?* Do this, and you'll never have a case of Monday morning angst again.

\- Embrace yourself in all your forms. Cancer taught me that we morph and change, sometimes into versions unrecognizable. It taught me that things change. That evolution is natural. It taught me that you do not always need to be the best version of yourself, all the time. It is okay to be tired, angry, sad, bald, or even just ten pounds too heavy. There are many versions of you, and that is the best part.

\- Lose yourself, whenever you can, wherever you can. Cancer made me realize that I wasn't in control. That I was never in control. Life is out of my control. There is no plan that can be made, and there is no map. We are all just trying to figure it out. We are all survivors. And that adventure, in itself, is wild, torrential, and *beautiful.* Give in to it. Go get lost.

So, that happened. Sickness happened. Change happened. Awareness happened. Transformation happened. *Life* happened.

I wonder what happens next.

ACKNOWLEDGMENTS

I would like to express my very great appreciation for all of those that helped me through the year that cancer happened. The medical oncology team at New York-Presbyterian/Weill Cornell Medical Center and all the specialists, experts, researchers, nurses, and staff dedicated to the Weill Cornell Lymphoma Program. The nurses and staff at the Hematology/ Oncology Infusion Center at Weill Cornell. Kepal N. Patel, M.D., and the staff at New York University Langone Hospital and the New York University Endocrine Surgery Associates. Penelope McDonnell, N.D., at Naturopathic Partners.

A very special thanks to my wonderful, witty, patient, and generous friends, without whom I would have cracked. And to my family, who are the best part of me.

I would like to thank the following people for their assistance in publishing the book. Stephanie Gunning, editor and publishing consultant. Graphic designer Gus Yoo.

ABOUT THE AUTHOR

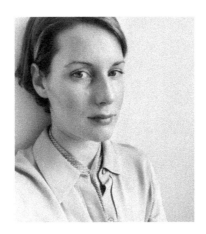

CC Webster is a former advertising industry executive who specialized in pharmaceutical healthcare advertising for an agency in New York City. Diagnosed with lymphoma at age twenty-nine, she began her course through treatment, which led to the exploration and discovery of health, happiness, and herself.

From first diagnosis to current remission, CC has combined eastern and western medicine to wage a war on cancer and support her body throughout its fight. The result has been the discovery of a healthier self, a happier self, a new self.

Due to the success of her integrative and explorative approach, CC now shares her story in hopes of helping others become their happiest, healthiest, optimal selves, and at the very least, invite some humor along the way.